D1561028

Attention Disorders After Right Brain Damage

Paolo Bartolomeo

Attention Disorders After Right Brain Damage

Living in Halved Worlds

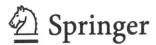 Springer

Paolo Bartolomeo, MD, PhD
Brain and Spine Institute
Hôpital de la Salpêtrière
Institut national de la santé et de la
recherche médicale (INSERM)
Paris
France

Department of Psychology
Catholic University
Milan
Italy

ISBN 978-1-4471-5648-2   ISBN 978-1-4471-5649-9   (eBook)
DOI 10.1007/978-1-4471-5649-9
Springer London Heidelberg New York Dordrecht

Library of Congress Control Number: 2013957355

Springer is part of Springer Science+Business Media (www.springer.com)

Foreword

Among the many mysteries of the human brain, one remains the most blatant but least unveiled. Namely, our brain (but also that of other species) is made of two distinct, grossly symmetrical parts – the right and left hemispheres – which entertain rich interconnections but also substantial independence and even remarkable specialization (perhaps unlike any other species). Such division of labor contrasts with our subjective sense of unity in thoughts, intentions, perceptions, or memories. This is patent when looking straight ahead in our central visual field: although its representation in occipital visual cortex is split in the midline across the two hemispheres, several centimeters apart, we experience no perceptible discontinuity. This unity of bilaterally distributed neural activities also occurs for our bodily sensations and actions, be it when we scratch our belly across the midline or play the piano with two hands, and even more so when we apprehend and explore space around us.

Because this unity is so powerful and feels so natural, it often takes a lesion in brain circuits to make the fundamental hemispheric division of our brain more apparent and unfortunately troublesome for brain-damaged patients. Such revealing nature of clinical disorders of cognition and behavior is precisely what makes neuropsychology a unique and irreplaceable approach to understanding the brain and mind. Further, besides basic neuroscience knowledge, in clinical practice, accurate recognition of deficits specific to lesions affecting one or the other hemisphere is a major step for correct diagnosis. For example, neuropsychological signs of right brain dysfunction in a patient with word naming difficulties may disclose unsuspected bilateral or multifocal disease such as dementia or multiple sclerosis and thus require totally different clinical investigations.

By providing a comprehensive overview of right brain functions and dysfunctions, masterfully assembled in a coherent neurocognitive framework, the present volume by Paolo Bartolomeo provides a compelling testimonial for both the clinical and scientific importance of pathologies of the right hemisphere. Traditional neurology terminology has qualified the right side of the human brain as being the "minor" hemisphere, as opposed to the "dominance" of the left for language and manual dexterity. However, as reviewed in this book, the right hemisphere is associated with a very rich set of functions, many of which actually touch the highest among high-level cognitive abilities. Not only attention and awareness are crucially dependent on right hemispheric networks but also space representation, navigation, mental flexibility and inhibitory control, mathematics, face recognition, emotion, music, as well as body ownership and key aspects of self-experience – all are deeply rooted in nonverbal integrative processes mediated by the (so-called) "minor" right hemisphere. These abilities seem in many ways as complex as language or dexterous hand movements, if not more. Moreover, their impairment leads to severe handicaps in everyday life. Thus, given the many essential functions subtended by the right hemisphere, one may wonder whether neurologists from another civilization (perhaps more attentive to nonverbal abilities) would have conceived this hemisphere as actually being the dominant one, generating the substance of sensory and experiential phenomena that may then be passed on to the subordinate left hemisphere for speech and hand motor outputs. At the very least, in a democratic brain, the right hemisphere should certainly be treated equally to the left and not put in a minority position.

Paolo Bartolomeo therefore does full justice to the right hemisphere by devoting this new book to the sophisticated cognitive apparatus of this significant half of the brain and its deficiencies following various pathologies. The book also cogently dissects the intricate relationships of right hemispheric disorders with attention and space. A major focus is put on the neglect syndrome and related disabilities, in keeping with the high frequency of such symptoms after right brain damage and their key interest for neuropsychology and cognitive neuroscience of attention processes. The successive chapters provide a complete and articulate coverage of several facets of attentional disorders, from the description of various behavioral phenomena through to the analysis of the underlying cerebral substrates. This systematic review is provided in a very fluid and synthetic manner, revealing the encyclopedic knowledge and critical perspective of the author. Throughout the book, a remarkable quality is the attempt to relate clinical observations to rigorous experimental measures, link them to precise cognitive mechanisms and neuroanatomical substrates, and integrate these data with current theoretical frameworks derived from neuroscience research in both human and nonhuman primates. In this process, the author portrays a compelling model of functional brain networks made of distributed and interactive regional nodes, whose functioning is dynamically shaped by attentional states and differentially impaired by pathology. This perspective does not only help provide a valuable mechanistic account for neglect and other neuropsychological disorders in right-brain-damaged patients but also open useful perspectives for remediation strategies. As such, the book will offer a unique resource for clinicians and students eager to learn about neuropsychology and its foundations in more basic brain sciences, while it will also supply researchers from various fields with a precious source of references and stimulating new ideas, organized with a well-structured manner and critical thinking.

In sum, by being a skilled clinician as well as an incisive researcher who made key contributions to current scientific knowledge on attention and neglect, and by craftily combining this personal experience with a broader neuroscience literature, Paolo Bartolomeo gives us here an admirable tutorial that clearly demonstrates (and explains) the major functions and disorders of the (not so) minor hemisphere.

Geneva, Switzerland   Patrik Vuilleumier

Preface and Acknowledgments

In a neurological ward, it is frequent to come upon patients who look at objects on their right side with intense interest, while paying no attention to what happens on their left. Left visual neglect is a dramatic but often overlooked consequence of right hemisphere damage, usually of vascular origin, but also resulting from other causes, such as neurodegenerative conditions. Patients do not eat from the left part of their dish, they bump their wheelchair into obstacles situated on their left side, and have a tendency to look at right-sided details as soon as a visual scene deploys, as if their attention were "magnetically" attracted to these details. They are usually unaware of their deficits (anosognosia) and often obstinately deny being hemiplegic. Patients with left brain damage may also show signs of contralesional, right-sided neglect, but much more rarely and usually in a less severe form. Diagnosis is important because neglect predicts poor functional outcome in stroke. Moreover, effective rehabilitation strategies are becoming available, and there are promising possibilities for pharmacological treatments.

At least since the time of Paul Broca's famous statement that "we speak with the left hemisphere," the role of the right, "nonspeaking" hemisphere has been the object of questioning. After decades of limited interest in the then called "nondominant" or "minor" hemisphere, beginning in the second half of the twentieth century (Brain 1941; McFie et al. 1950), a wealth of research has burgeoned in subjects dealing with deficits resulting from right hemisphere lesions, especially in the domain of visual neglect. Clinically, damage to the right hemisphere can lead to substantial levels of handicap and disability, which are probably even more severe and long-lasting than those occurring after lesions of similar volume and localization in the left hemisphere (Denes et al. 1982). For example, as Ennio De Renzi stated in his seminal book on spatial cognition (De Renzi 1982), "Unilateral spatial neglect after right hemispheric lesions has equal clinical and scientific importance to language disorders after left lesions."

Nevertheless, it is fair to say that work on right brain deficits has had a much lesser impact on clinical practice than research on aphasias or other neuropsychological consequences of left hemisphere damage. Perhaps as a result of this state of affairs, functional scores used in clinical settings (e.g., the Mini Mental State

Examination or the National Institutes of Health Stroke Scale Scores) are heavily biased towards language and consequently underestimate the functional impairment resulting from right hemisphere lesions (Fink et al. 2002). Another consequence of the general lack of knowledge of deficits related to right hemisphere damage is that minor strokes in the right hemisphere are likely to pass completely undetected, thus exposing patients to the risk of more severe lesions in the absence of diagnosis and consequent secondary prevention.

The idea for this book issued from the observance of this state of affairs and the frank admission that knowledge, albeit incomplete, of the clinical and neuropsychological consequences of right hemisphere lesions may be better integrated into everyday clinical practice. This book attempts to provide an overview of attentional impairments in right-brain-damaged patients from both clinical and neuroscientific perspectives and aims at offering a comprehensive, if succinct, treatment of topics such as body and perceptual awareness and visual neglect.

The first chapter outlines some current ideas about the attention systems and how they are implemented in the human brain. Chapter 2 is devoted to some unexpected instances of hemispheric asymmetries in sensorimotor deficits, whereby hemianopia and hemianesthesia can apparently occur more often after right than after left brain damage, and to disturbances of perceptual awareness (extinction) and of gaze control. Attention deficits have most certainly a role in these disorders. Chapter 3 explores some neuropsychological consequences of lesions to the right hemisphere of the brain, in particular those relative to the patients' awareness and control of their own bodies. At the present time it is unclear whether and how these disorders relate to attention processes, but some of them, such as anosognosia, are of considerable clinical importance due to their consequences on patients' functional outcome.

Chapter 4 concerns unilateral spatial neglect, the most important clinical syndrome resulting from right brain damage, in its clinical diagnostic aspects. Beyond its clinical importance, neglect has fostered a wealth of research efforts in cognitive neuroscience during the last decades. Chapter 5 reviews some experimental variants of clinical paradigms, developed in order to better understand the mechanisms of this complex condition. The (provisional) conclusions of these ongoing endeavors are outlined in Chap. 6.

The following Chap. 7 is dedicated to the anatomical underpinnings of neglect signs and to the relations between the localization of the lesions producing neglect and the attention networks in the right hemisphere. These chapters mainly relate to focal brain damage such as that resulting from vascular strokes or tumors. However, with the increase of life expectancy in Western countries, neurodegenerative conditions such as Alzheimer's disease are becoming a growing concern in public health because their frequency and severity increase with age. Importantly also, patients suffering from these diseases frequently display attention disorders, often related to predominantly right hemisphere degeneration. This relatively unfamiliar issue is the focus of Chap. 8. Finally, several promising lines of treatment have been proposed for attention disorder of neurological origin (especially spatial neglect), from behavioral techniques to physical or even pharmacological interventions. Chapter 9 outlines these therapeutic protocols, from the rehabilitation techniques which are already common practice to more experimental treatments such as transcranial magnetic stimulation or drugs.

The nature of the disorders outlined in this book, as well as the identity and functioning of the corresponding "normal" cognitive abilities, is currently the object of hot debate and constitutes some of the most controversial topics in cognitive neurology and neuroscience. To simplify, we are not sure whether we hold the right theoretical instruments in order to interpret such mysterious phenomena as conscious perception, bottom-up and top-down attention, bodily awareness, emotional responses to disease, and so on. This book does not pretend to solve these mysteries; instead, it aims at providing a guide to clinical facts which are hard to find described together in a single source. It is intended for an essentially clinical readership.

Some of the topics which are not discussed in this book include important instances of neuropsychological deficits resulting from right hemisphere damage, with a possibly less direct link to attention processes. These include deficits of face processing, or prosopagnosia (De Renzi et al. 1994), of emotional processing (Gainotti 2012), of social skills (Corbetta et al. 2008), apraxia for dressing (Hier et al. 1983), and the acquired inability to discriminate voices, or phonagnosia (Van Lancker et al. 1988). For essentially practical purposes, the scope of this book is restricted to neurological disorders acquired in adult life; this leaves out important topics such as the attention-deficit hyperactivity disorder (ADHD), to which right hemispheric dysfunctions might well contribute (Castellanos and Tannock 2002).

The guidance and help of my mentor and "maestro" Guido Gainotti has been essential to me for decades, ever since I was assigned my MD thesis on visual neglect in Rome. This book is no exception.

Over the last two decades, I had the chance to collaborate with a number of brilliant students, some of whom are now talented co-workers, such as Katia Andrade, Alexia Bourgeois, Clémence Bourlon, Francesca Ciaraffa, Caroline Decaix, Federica Rastelli, Michel Thiebaut de Schotten, Monica Toba, and Marika Urbanski. Their hard work and good humor have been critical antecedents of this book. Important contributions to the research and writing of this volume also came from many colleagues and friends, including Philippe Azouvi, Anne-Catherine Bachoud-Lévi, Marco Catani, Patrick Cavanagh, Ana B. Chica, Sylvie Chokron, Gianfranco Dalla Barba, Patrizia D'Erme, Fabrizio Doricchi, Hugues Duffau, Raffaella (Lara) Migliaccio, Juan Lupiáñez, Orazio Miglino, Gilles Rode, Eric Siéroff, Antoni Valero-Cabré, and Patrik Vuilleumier.

Special thanks are due to Anne Petrov, who not only streamlined the English of this work but also the author's thinking in many instances. I am grateful to Joanna Bolesworth of Springer UK for her support, assistance, and incessant but always kind exhortations to go ahead with writing. The writing of this book was supported by the European Union FP6 and ANR project eraNET-NEURON BEYONDVIS and by a Translational Research grant from the Assistance Publique-Hôpitaux de Paris (AP-HP).

This book is dedicated to the author's beloved four girls: Lida, Francesca, Teresa, and Caterina.

References

Brain RW. Visual disorientation with special reference to lesion of the right brain hemisphere. Brain. 1941;64:244–72.

Castellanos FX, Tannock R. Neuroscience of attention-deficit/hyperactivity disorder: the search for endophenotypes. Nat Rev Neurosci. 2002;3:617–28.

Corbetta M, Patel G, Shulman GL. The reorienting system of the human brain: from environment to theory of mind. Neuron. 2008;58:306–24.

Denes G, Semenza C, Stoppa E, Lis A. Unilateral spatial neglect and recovery from hemiplegia: a follow-up study. Brain. 1982;105:543–52.

De Renzi E. Disorders of space elaboration and cognition. New York: Wiley; 1982.

De Renzi E, Perani D, Carlesimo GA, Silveri MC, Fazio F. Prosopagnosia can be associated with damage confined to the right hemisphere – an MRI and PET study and a review of the literature. Neuropsychologia. 1994;32:893–902.

Fink JN, Selim MH, Kumar S, Silver B, Linfante I, Caplan LR, Schlaug G. Is the association of National Institutes of Health Stroke Scale scores and acute magnetic resonance imaging stroke volume equal for patients with right- and left-hemisphere ischemic stroke? Stroke. 2002;33:954–58.

Gainotti G. Unconscious processing of emotions and the right hemisphere. Neuropsychologia. 2012;50:205–18.

Hier DB, Mondlock J, Caplan LR. Behavioral abnormalities after right hemisphere stroke. Neurology. 1983;33:337–44.

McFie J, Piercy MF, Zangwill OL. Visual spatial agnosia associated with lesions of the right hemisphere. Brain. 1950;73:167–90.

Van Lancker DR, Cummings JL, Kreiman J, Dobkin BH. Phonagnosia: a dissociation between familiar and unfamiliar voices. Cortex. 1988;24:195–209.

Abbreviations

ACC	Anterior cingulate cortex
AD	Alzheimer's disease
ARE	Attention repulsion effect
BA	Brodmann area
BOLD	Blood oxygenation level dependent
CBS	Corticobasal syndrome
DAN	Dorsal attentional network
DTI	Diffusion tensor imaging
EBA	Extra-striate body area
ERP	Evoked potential response
FBA	Fusiform body area
FEF	Frontal eye field
FTD	Frontotemporal dementia
IFOF	Inferior fronto-occipital fasciculus
ILF	Inferior longitudinal fasciculus
IOR	Inhibition of return
IPL	Inferior parietal lobule
IPS	Intraparietal sulcus
ISI	Interstimulus interval
MRI	Magnetic resonance imaging
PCA	Posterior cerebral atrophy
PFC	Prefrontal cortex
PPC	Posterior parietal cortex
REMs	Rapid eye movements
SLF	Superior longitudinal fasciculus
SOA	Stimulus-onset asynchrony
SPL	Superior parietal lobule
SWM	Spatial working memory
tDCS	Transcranial direct current stimulation

TMS	Transcranial magnetic stimulation
TPJ	Temporoparietal junction
VAN	Ventral attentional network
VLSM	Voxel-based lesion–symptom mapping

Contents

Chapter 1
The Attention Systems of the Human Brain

Keywords Selection • Alertness • Vigilance • Control • Endogenous attention •
Exogenous attention • Inhibition of return • Frontoparietal networks

We live in an environment cluttered with a multitude of objects. To behave in a
coherent and goal-driven way, we need to select stimuli appropriate to our goals.
On the other hand, because of capacity limitations, we must be capable of ignoring other less important objects. Thus, in a sense, objects in the world compete
for recruiting our attention in order to be the focus of our subsequent behavior.
Neural mechanisms of attention resolve this competition by taking into account
both the agent's goals and the salience of the sensorial stimuli (Desimone and
Duncan 1995). Thus, attention to external information can help the agent select
locations in space, points in time, or modality-specific input (Chun et al. 2011).
Other attention processes select, modulate, and maintain internally generated
information, such as task rules, responses, long-term memory, or working memory (Chun et al. 2011).

Attention and its neural correlates are not unitary phenomena; they can be better
understood as a heterogeneous, if interacting, set of processes. For example,
Parasuraman (1998) identified at least three independent but interacting components of attention: (1) selection, that is, mechanisms determining more extensive
processing of some input rather than others; (2) vigilance, the capacity of sustaining
attention over time; (3) control, the ability of planning and coordinating different
activities (Table 1.1).

In sum, attention must allow an organism to successfully cope with a continu-
ously changing external and internal environment, while maintaining its goals.
This flexibility calls for mechanisms that (a) allow for the processing of novel,
unexpected events, which could be either advantageous or dangerous, in order to
respond appropriately with either approaching or avoidance behavior, and (b)
allow for the maintenance of finalized behavior despite distracting events (Allport
1989). For example, attention can be directed at an object in space either in a relatively reflexive way (e.g., when a honking car attracts the attention of a pedestrian)

P. Bartolomeo, *Attention Disorders After Right Brain Damage*,
DOI 10.1007/978-1-4471-5649-9_1, © Springer-Verlag London 2014

Table 1.1 A schematic taxonomy of attention processes and of their anatomical bases. Note the functional and neural overlap between attentional capture (exogenous attention) and sustained (vigilant) attention

Type of attention	Function	Anatomy
Spatial selective attention	Orienting of attention to spatial locations and to objects in space	Bilateral DAN (SPL, IPS and dorsolateral PFC)
Stimulus-driven attentional capture	Processing of unexpected events	Right hemisphere VAN (IPL, TPJ and ventrolateral PFC)
Sustained (vigilant) attention or tonic alertness	Rapid responses to external stimuli (independent of their spatial position)	Right hemisphere VAN, thalamic and brain stem nuclei (esp. locus coeruleus), ACC, anterior insula
Phasic alertness	Alertness externally generated by a warning signal	Vigilant attention network + left PFC and thalamus
Arousal	General wakefulness and responsiveness	Diffuse cortical projections from brain stem nuclei (basal forebrain, locus coeruleus, medial forebrain bundle, dorsal raphe nucleus).
Executive control	Monitoring and conflict solving	Dorsal ACC, dorsolateral PFC, right ventrolateral PFC (IFG)

or in a more controlled mode (e.g., when the pedestrian monitors the traffic light waiting for the "go" signal to appear). It is thereby plausible that different attention processes serve these two partially conflicting goals (Chica et al. 2013a). A traditional distinction in experimental psychology refers to more exogenous (or stimulus-dependent, bottom-up) processes for orienting attention to novel events (Yantis 1995), as opposed to more endogenous (or strategy-driven, top-down) orienting processes, which would be responsible for directing the organism's attention towards relevant targets despite the presence of distractors in the environment (LaBerge et al. 2000).

1.1 Spatial Selective Attention

The concept of spatial selective attention refers operationally to the advantage in speed and accuracy of processing for objects lying in attended regions of space as compared to objects located in non-attended regions (Posner 1980).

When several events compete for limited processing capacity and control of behavior, attention selection may resolve the competition. In their influential neurocognitive model of selective attention, Desimone and Duncan (1995) proposed that competition is biased towards some stimuli over others by neural attention processes on the basis of the organisms' goals and of the sensory properties of the objects, thereby giving priority to some objects over others.

1.1.1 Manual Response Time Paradigms

A subset of these selective attention processes deals with objects in space. In eco-logical settings outside the laboratory, agents usually orient towards important stim-uli by turning their gaze, head, and trunk towards their spatial location. This is done in order to align the stimulus with the part of the sensory surface with the highest resolution (e.g., the retinal fovea) (Di Ferdinando et al. 2007). This allows further perceptual processing of the detected stimulus, for example, its classification as a useful or as a dangerous object. Even very simple artificial organisms display ori-enting behavior when their processing resources are insufficient to process the whole visual scene in parallel (Di Ferdinando et al. 2007). However, attention can also be oriented in space without eye movements, via so-called "covert" orienting (Posner 1980).

Posner and his co-workers developed a manual response time (RT) paradigm to study the covert orienting of attention. Subjects are presented with three horizon-tally arranged boxes (Fig. 1.1).

They fixate the central box and respond by pressing a key to a target (an aster-isk) appearing in one of two lateral boxes. The target is preceded by a cue indicat-ing one of the two lateral boxes. Cues can be either central (an arrow or another symbol presented in the central box) or peripheral (a brief brightening of one peripheral box). Valid cues correctly predict the box in which the target will appear, whereas invalid cues indicate the wrong box. Normal subjects usually show a cue validity effect consisting in faster RTs and increased accuracy for valid cue-target trials than for invalid trials (but see the phenomenon of inhibition of return described below). This suggests that the cue prompts an attention orient-ing towards the cued location, which speeds up the processing of targets appear-ing in that region and slows down responses to targets appearing in other locations.

In this paradigm, it is often the case that a large majority (e.g., 80 %) of cues are valid; in this case, cues are said to be informative of the future position of the tar-get. Alternatively, cues may be non-informative, when targets can appear with equal probabilities in the cued or in the uncued location. Peripheral non-informa-tive cues attract attention automatically or exogenously. This exogenous attention shift (revealed by a cue validity effect) is typically observed only for short stimu-lus-onset asynchronies (SOAs) between cue and target. For SOAs longer than ~300 ms, uncued targets evoke faster responses than cued targets (Posner and Cohen 1984; Maylor and Hockey 1985; Rafal and Henik 1994). This phenomenon is known as inhibition of return (IOR) (Posner et al. 1985; Bartolomeo and Lupiáñez 2006) and is often interpreted as reflecting a mechanism which promotes the exploration of the visual scene by inhibiting repeated orientations towards the same locations (Posner and Cohen 1984; Klein 2000; but see Berlucchi 2006). Exogenous, or stimulus-dependent, and endogenous, or strategy-driven, mecha-nisms of attention orienting are thus qualitatively different, though highly interac-tive, processes (Chica et al. 2013a). An interesting property of exogenous orienting

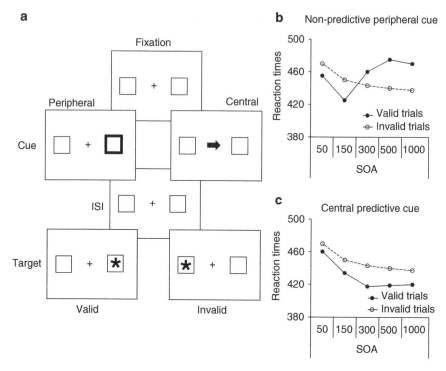

Fig. 1.1 (**a**) Illustration of a typical Posner paradigm (From Chica et al. 2013a). Targets can be preceded by either peripheral cues (*left*) or central cues (*right*). (**b**) Typical response time results (in milliseconds) observed when peripheral non-predictive cues precede targets at different SOAs (stimulus-onset asynchronies, the time intervals between the onset of the cue, and the onset of the target). Reaction times are faster for valid vs. invalid trials at short SOAs, but the effect reverses at SOAs longer than 300 ms, demonstrating an IOR effect. (**c**) Typical response time results observed when central predictive cues precede targets at different SOAs. Reaction times are faster for valid vs. invalid trials, and the effect is sustained even at the longest SOA. ISI (inter-stimulus interval) is the time interval between the end of the cue and the beginning of the target (Reproduced from Chica et al. (2013a). © 2013, with permission from Elsevier)

of attention is that it does not remain focused on the stimulated spatial position but tends to spread to the whole perceptual object presented in that region (Egly et al. 1994; Macquistan 1997).

1.1.2 Anatomical Brain Structures and Networks of Spatial Attention

Today, we know a fair amount of detailed information about the anatomy, functions, dynamics, and pathological dysfunctions of the brain networks that subserve the orienting of gaze and attention in the human brain. Here, we describe some of the

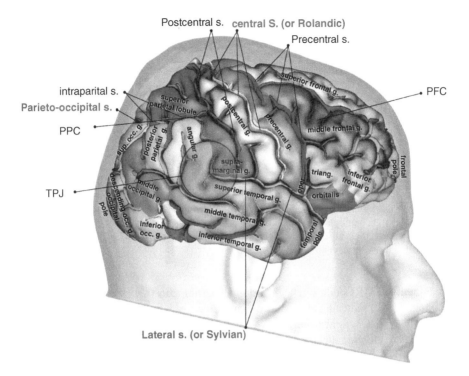

Fig. 1.2 3D reconstruction of the lateral surface of the right hemisphere. *G* gyrus, *s* sulcus. The prefrontal cortex (*PFC*) lies anterior to the precentral gyrus; the posterior parietal cortex (*PPC*) lies posterior to the postcentral gyrus. The inferior parietal lobule is composed of the angular gyrus and of the supramarginal gyrus. The temporoparietal junction (*TPJ*) comprises the caudal part of the superior temporal gyrus and the ventral part of the IPL (Modified from Catani and Thiebaut de Schotten (2012). © 2012. Reproduced with permission of Oxford University Press (www.oup.com))

observations based on neurophysiological techniques in the monkey or functional magnetic resonance imaging (MRI) in humans to pinpoint the anatomical structures and networks which are activated during the performance of attention-related functions. Important components of these networks include the dorsolateral prefrontal cortex (PFC) and the posterior parietal cortex (PPC) (Fig. 1.2).

Physiological studies indicate that these two structures show interdependence of neural activity and thus compose a functional frontoparietal network. In the monkey, analogous PPC and PFC areas show coordinated activity when the animal selects a visual stimulus as a saccade target (Buschman and Miller 2007). Importantly, PFC and PPC show distinctive dynamics and seem to use two different "languages" when attention is drawn by the stimulus (such as in bottom-up or exogenous orienting) or when it is directed by more strategy-driven (top-down or endogenous) goals. In particular, bottom-up signals appear first in the parietal cortex and are characterized by an increase of frontoparietal coherence in the gamma band (25–100 Hz), whereas top-down signals emerge first in the frontal cortex and tend to synchronize in the beta band (12–30 Hz) (Buschman and Miller 2007).

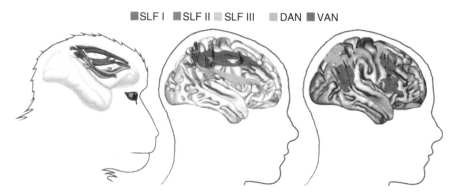

Fig. 1.3 Frontoparietal networks in the monkey (*left*, from Schmahmann and Pandya 2006) and in the human right hemisphere (*middle*, from Thiebaut de Schotten et al. 2011). *Right*: attentional networks in the right hemisphere according to Corbetta and Shulman (2002) (Figure as originally published in Bartolomeo et al. (2012))

Functional MRI studies in healthy human participants (reviewed by Corbetta and Shulman 2002) indicate the existence of multiple frontoparietal networks for spatial attention (Fig. 1.3, right panel).

A dorsal attentional network (DAN), composed of the intraparietal sulcus (IPS)/ superior parietal lobule and the frontal eye field (FEF)/dorsolateral PFC, shows increased blood-oxygenation-level dependent (BOLD) responses during the orienting period. Functional MRI also demonstrated a ventral attentional network (VAN), which includes the temporoparietal junction (TPJ) and the ventral PFC (inferior and middle frontal gyri), and shows increased BOLD responses when participants have to respond to targets presented in unexpected locations.

Thus, the VAN is considered important for detecting unexpected but behaviorally relevant events. Importantly, the DAN is bilateral and symmetrical, whereas the VAN is strongly lateralized to the right hemisphere. According to Singh-Curry and Husain (2009), the VAN is not only dedicated to salience detection in a stimulus-driven way but is also responsible for maintaining attention on goals or task demands, which is a top-down process (see Sect. 1.2 below). In support of this proposal, functional MRI has suggested a role for the inferior frontal junction (parts of BA 9, 44, 6) in mediating interactions between bottom-up and top-down attention (Asplund et al. 2010). Furthermore, TPJ, the caudal node of the VAN, demonstrates increased BOLD response for behaviorally relevant distractors, but not for nonrelevant but highly salient ones (Indovina and Macaluso 2007).

These anatomical regions are likely to be distinguishable as distinct clusters with different cytoarchitectonic structure, white matter connections, and functional properties. For example, reorienting to unexpected (invalid) targets and the processing of competition exerted by distractors may implicate different portions of the PPC. In a functional MRI study which took into account the cytoarchitectonic subdivisions of the PPC (Gillebert et al. 2013), areas hIP1 and hIP3 in the IPS (Fig. 1.4) demonstrated an effect of competition, whereas area PF in the supramarginal gyrus

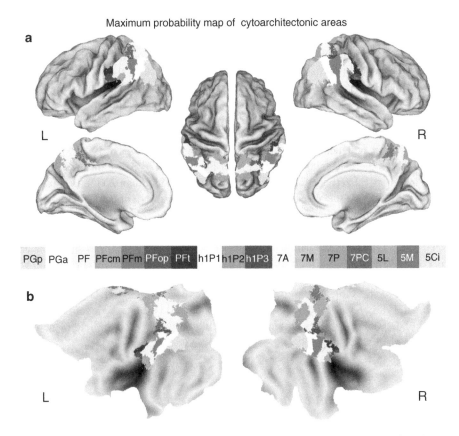

Fig. 1.4 Maximum probability maps of cytoarchitectonic areas in parietal cortex projected onto (**a**) a surface rendering of the brain (lateral, medial and dorsal view) and (**b**) on the flattened brain surface. *L* left hemisphere, *R* right hemisphere (Reproduced from Gillebert et al. (2013). © 2013, with permission from Elsevier)

of the right hemisphere showed an invalidity effect in the absence of competition effect. Other areas, such as PFm in the supramarginal gyrus and PGa in the angular gyrus, showed both an invalidity and a competition effect.

Importantly and not surprisingly given the functional neuroimaging evidence of frontoparietal attentional networks, PFC and PPC are directly and extensively interconnected by anatomical white matter tracts. In particular, studies in the monkey brain have identified three distinct frontoparietal long-range branches of the superior longitudinal fasciculus (SLF) on the basis of cortical terminations and course (Petrides and Pandya 1984; Schmahmann and Pandya 2006) (see Fig. 1.3, left panel). Recent evidence from advanced in vivo tractography techniques and postmortem dissections suggests that a similar architecture exists in the human brain (Thiebaut de Schotten et al. 2011) (Fig. 1.3, middle panel). In humans, the most dorsal branch (SLF I) originates from Brodmann areas (BA) 5 and 7 and projects to BA 8, 9, and 32. The middle pathway (SLF II) originates in BA 39 and 40 within the inferior parietal lobule (IPL) and reaches prefrontal BA 8 and 9. The most ventral pathway (SLF III) originates in BA 40 and terminates in BA 44, 45, and 47. These results are consistent with the functional MRI evidence on attentional networks mentioned above. In particular, the SLF III connects the cortical nodes of the VAN, whereas the DAN is connected by the human homologue of SLF I. The SLF II connects the parietal component of the VAN to the prefrontal component of the DAN, thus allowing direct communication between ventral and dorsal attentional networks.

Anatomical evidence is in good agreement with asymmetries of BOLD response during functional MRI, showing larger right-hemisphere response for the VAN and more symmetrical activity for the DAN (Corbetta and Shulman 2002), because the SLF III (connecting the VAN) is anatomically larger in the right hemisphere than in the left hemisphere, whereas the SLF I (connecting the DAN) is more symmetrically organized (Thiebaut de Schotten et al. 2011). SLF II also tends to be right-lateralized, but with substantial interindividual differences. The lateralization of SLF II is strongly correlated to behavioral signs of right-hemisphere specialization for visuospatial attention such as pseudoneglect online bisection, i.e., small leftward deviations of the subjective midline produced by normal individuals (Bowers and Heilman 1980; Jewell and McCourt 2000; Toba 2011), and asymmetries in the speed of detection of events presented in the right or in the left hemifield (Thiebaut de Schotten et al. 2011).

1.1.3 Spatial Attention and Visual Awareness

Introspection suggests that when we attend to an object or part of a scene we become aware of it. Removing attention from the object makes it fade from awareness. Although there seems to be a consensus regarding the fact that some level of general alertness (see Sect. 1.2 below) is needed in order to attain conscious perception (Robertson et al. 1998; Dehaene and Changeux 2011; Kusnir et al. 2011), the relationship between spatial attention and conscious perception has proven difficult to explore empirically (see Chica and Bartolomeo 2012, for review).

Several lines of evidence support the hypothesis that some form of attention is necessary for conscious perception (Posner 1994). A classical example is observed the inattentional blindness paradigm, where salient changes in the features of visual stimuli are missed when unattended (Mack and Rock 1998), even when stimuli are presented at the fovea. In one of the most striking examples of the influence of attention on visual awareness (Simons and Chabris 1999), normal participants were asked to view a movie clip wherein two groups of people wearing black or white T-shirts made basketball passes. Participants had to count ball passes made by members of one of the teams while ignoring those made by the other team. Unexpectedly, a character dressed up as a gorilla crossed the visual scene during the ball passes. Around half of the participants typically failed to see the gorilla. Presumably, their attention prevented them from noticing the strange and perceptually conspicuous event because attention was fully engaged in the difficult task of actively following a dynamic scene (the ball passes performed by one team) while selecting out another (the ball passes made by the other team). Thus, distracting attention can prevent highly salient items from entering awareness in normal individuals. These counter-intuitive findings, along with many others (reviewed by Chica and Bartolomeo 2012), stress the crucial importance of spatial attention, and its modulation, for the building of our conscious experience.

Concerning the neural bases of such interactions between spatial attention and visual awareness, functional MRI results obtained by using variants of the Posner paradigm (Chica and Bartolomeo 2012) indicate an important role of functionally connected frontoparietal attention networks across the two cerebral hemispheres. Functional MRI signals were recorded while participants responded to near-threshold stimuli preceded by peripheral cues. Functional connectivity analyses during the orienting period (i.e., during the processing of the attentional cue, before the target was presented) demonstrated that activity in a right-lateralized frontopa-rietal network, including superior and inferior parietal lobes, the left FEF, the right insula, and right IFG (Fig. 1.5), was tightly correlated to spatial attention and con-scious reports. In particular, a strong functional connection between right IPL and

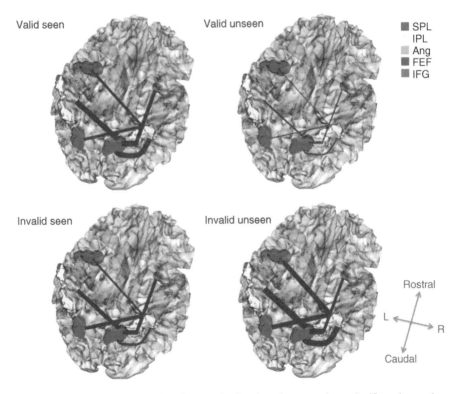

Fig. 1.5 Schematic depiction of the frontoparietal regions demonstrating a significant interaction between cue validity (valid or invalid cues) and reportability of the future target (seen, unseen) in the fMRI experiment by Chica et al. (2013b). *Line thickness* represents the strength of the beta correlation value between two regions. *SPL* superior parietal lobule, *IPL* inferior parietal lobule, *ANG* angular gyrus, *FEF* frontal eye field, *IFG* inferior frontal gyrus (Reproduced from Chica et al. (2013b). © 2013, with permission from Oxford University Press)

left FEF emerged, suggesting that interhemispheric cooperation between the right VAN and the left DAN may have an important role in the interaction between spatial orienting and conscious perception.

Strong coupling within this bihemispheric network correlated with conscious reports when targets were presented at the attended location; however, the same coupling correlated instead with "unseen" reports when targets were presented at unattended locations. Frontoparietal interactions can therefore be primed by attentional processes, thus increasing the likelihood of conscious reports. Evidence of interaction between spatial attention and consciousness was observed in frontoparietal regions, but not in lower level visual areas, which is consistent with reports of neural dissociations between spatial attention and visual awareness in the visual cortex (Wyart and Tallon-Baudry 2008).

1.1.4 Attention and Visual Perception

1.1.4.1 Cortical Streams of Visual Processing

According to an influential model (Mishkin et al. 1983), visual information processed in the primary visual cortex (or striate cortex, see Fig. 2.1) follows two major pathways in the macaque brain. A dorsal cortical visual stream, concerned with visually guided movements in space (Goodale and Milner 1992), but also overlapping in part with the attention systems, reaches the IPL and the dorsolateral PFC. A ventral cortical visual stream, important for perceptual identification, projects from the occipital striate cortex to the inferior temporal cortex, with a further projection from the inferior temporal cortex to the ventral prefrontal cortex (Fig. 1.6).

More recently, the concept of dorsal visual stream has been refined by the identification of several pathways emerging from the dorsal stream that consist of projections to the prefrontal and premotor cortices (Rizzolatti and Matelli 2003) and a further projection to the medial temporal lobe (Kravitz et al. 2011). Also the ventral visual stream has recently been subdivided into several components, and the original hypothesis of a serial mode of processing from V1 to the inferior temporal cortex has now been revised to include more complex interactions, both feed-forward and feedback (Kravitz et al. 2013).

Indeed, the anatomy of long-range white matter tracts in these regions does suggest that both the dorsal and ventral streams can be further divided into distinct components. As mentioned before, there are at least three major subdivisions of the parietofrontal superior longitudinal fasciculus (SLF), both in the monkey (Schmahmann and Pandya 2006) and in the human brain (Thiebaut de Schotten et al. 2011). Concerning the occipitotemporal pathway, several functional systems are starting to emerge in the monkey (Kravitz et al. 2013). Anatomically, two major systems have been identified in the human brain. They run along the Inferior Longitudinal Fasciculus (ILF) and the Inferior Fronto-Occipital Fasciculus (IFOF) (Catani et al. 2003) (Fig. 1.7).

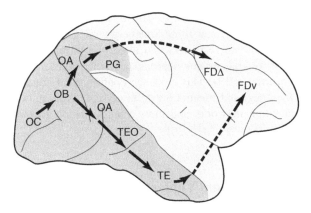

Fig. 1.6 The ventral and dorsal cortical visual streams in the macaque monkey. In the original description (Mishkin et al. 1983), the ventral stream is a multisynaptic pathway projecting from the striate cortex [cytoarchitectonic area (*OC*)] to area TE in the inferior temporal (IT) cortex, with a further projection from TE to the ventrolateral prefrontal region FDv. The dorsal pathway was described as a multisynaptic pathway projecting from the striate cortex to area PG in the inferior parietal lobule, with a further projection from PG to the dorsolateral prefrontal region FDΔ. The behavioral effects of lesions in monkeys suggested that the ventral pathway subserves object vision ("what"), whereas the dorsal pathway was characterized as supporting spatial vision ("where") (Reproduced from Kravitz et al. (2013). © 2013, with permission from Elsevier)

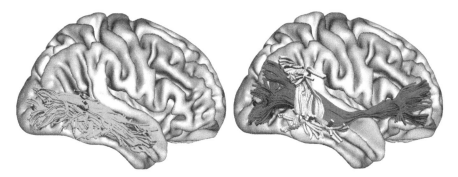

Fig. 1.7 Virtual in vivo dissection of the ILF (in *green*), the IFOF (in *red*), and the posterior segment of the superior longitudinal fasciculus (in *yellow*) (Reproduced from Thiebaut de Schotten et al. (2012). © 2012, with permission from Oxford University Press)

1.1.4.2   Attentional Modulations of Visual Perception

Attention influences in important ways not only the perception of near-threshold visual targets, as described in the previous section, but also the subjective perception of suprathreshold visual stimuli, for example, by increasing spatial resolution, i.e., the ability to discriminate between two nearby points in space (Carrasco et al. 2004).

Thus, neural activity in the ventral visual pathways is modulated by attentional processes (Moran and Desimone 1985; Sundberg et al. 2012). In particular, attention increases the neuronal responses and alters the profile and position of the receptive fields of ventral stream neurons near the attended location (Anton-Erxleben and Carrasco 2013). This evidence confirms that conscious perception emerges from the integrated functioning of large-scale brain networks, including frontoparietal attention networks and more ventral occipitotemporal streams of processing.

1.2   Sustained Attention, Vigilance, Alertness, Arousal

Another important component of attention, which does not necessarily involve selection, is the capacity to rapidly respond to external stimuli, whether or not accompanied by distractors. This aspect is often referred to as alertness, vigilant, or sustained attention, with a typical time span measured in seconds (Robertson and Garavan 2004).

The alerting system is believed to produce a general alert state that would be responsible for spreading attention over a broad area of space and is believed to be modulated by the locus coeruleus/norepinephrine system (Coull et al. 1999). A higher alert state allows for faster processing of information, independently of its spatial location (Fernandez-Duque and Posner 1997). We can voluntarily maintain our level of alertness over time, a function known as sustained attention, which involves the right PFC (Wilkins et al. 1987), the IPL, and subcortical structures (Sturm and Willmes 2001). Right frontoparietal systems can be important for modulating alertness, especially when alertness is to be generated in the absence of suitable external stimuli (Robertson and Garavan 2004). Thus, brain networks important for sustained attention include the PFC and PPC primarily in the right hemisphere (Pardo et al. 1991), with additional contribution from thalamic and brain stem nuclei (Sturm et al. 1999) (Fig. 1.8).

A "salience network" comprising the dorsal anterior cingulate cortex (ACC, Fig. 1.9) in the medial wall of the frontal lobe, the anterior insula, the thalamus, and the anterior PFC may be important to maintain tonic (sustained) alertness and facilitate stimulus detection (Sadaghiani et al. 2010). The ACC might thus constitute an important interface between the right frontoparietal cortical system and subcortical arousal mechanisms (Robertson and Garavan 2004).

In particular, the ACC could assume a key role in the modulation of alertness depending on task demands (Sturm et al. 1999, 2004; Mottaghy et al. 2006; Bartolomeo et al. 2008). The role of the ACC in the control of alertness is also underlined by the results of several neuroimaging studies focusing on this structure (review in Paus et al. 1998). This evidence shows that task difficulty was strongly correlated with activation peaks, especially in the supracallosal part of the ACC. More difficult tasks possibly call for an increased level of alertness and a higher activation of the brain stem catecholaminergic systems. Consistent with these notions, the ACC is densely connected to the noradrenergic (Gaspar et al. 1989) and

Fig. 1.8 Positron emission tomography activations for a task of sustained attention with visual stimuli (Sturm et al. 1999). The predominantly right hemisphere network encompasses the dorsolateral prefrontal cortex (*1*), the ACC (*2*), the inferior parietal cortex (*3*), the thalamus (*4*), and the pontomesencephalic tegmentum, possibly involving the locus coeruleus (*5*) (Reproduced from Sturm (2009), with the author's permission)

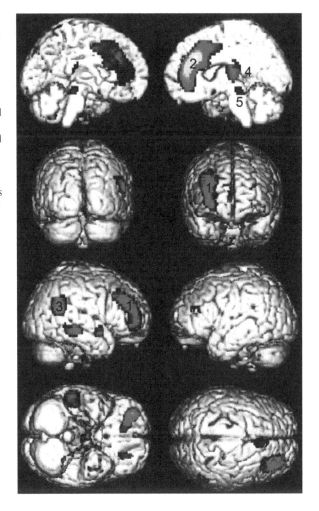

cholinergic (Mesulam et al. 1992) subcortical systems involved in the regulation of alertness (see also Sarter et al. 2001).

The alertness level can also be modulated experimentally by presenting warning signals that carry information about when, but not where, targets will appear. This is so-called phasic alertness. In addition to the mainly right-lateralized neural structures involved in sustained attention, phasic alertness is associated with activity in the left PFC and thalamus (Sturm and Willmes 2001).

Although sometimes used interchangeably with alertness, *arousal* should be referred to general wakefulness and responsiveness and related to slow circadian rhythms. Of particular importance for arousal are systems projecting to the cortex from the brain stem (Moruzzi and Magoun 1949), the cholinergic basal forebrain, the noradrenergic locus coeruleus (also implicated in alertness, see Aston-Jones and Cohen 2005), the dopaminergic medial forebrain bundle, and the serotoninergic dorsal raphe nucleus (Robertson and Garavan 2004).

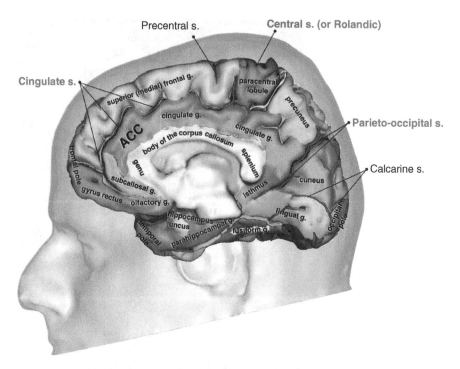

Fig. 1.9 3D reconstruction of the medial surface of the right hemisphere, showing the position of the anterior cingulate cortex (*ACC*). *G* gyrus, *s* sulcus (Modified from Catani and Thiebaut de Schotten (2012). © 2012. Reproduced with permission of Oxford University Press (www.oup.com))

1.3 Executive Control

A distinct dimension of attention processes involves executive control, which requires both monitoring and conflict solving, such as in the flankers task (Eriksen and Eriksen 1974), in the Stroop task (Stroop 1935) (Fig. 1.10), or in the Simon spatial compatibility effect (Lu and Proctor 1995). In these tasks, a prepotent but incorrect response must be inhibited to produce the correct response. For example, in the flanker task a target, such as an arrow, is flanked by two arrows of equal size on each side (left and right), pointing in the same direction as the central target (congruent trials) or in the opposite direction (incongruent trials). Participants are asked to respond as rapidly and as accurately as possible by pressing a right-sided button for right-sided targets and a left-sided button for left-sided targets. Responses are slower in the incongruent condition than in the congruent condition. In the Stroop color interference task (Stroop 1935), subjects must report the color of the ink of a word designating another color (e.g., *GREEN* printed in blue ink) or the same color (e.g., *RED* printed in red ink). Again, there is a slowing of performance in the nonmatching condition, which is believed to result from the interference from the prepotent but incorrect automatic response (reading the word) over the less automatic color naming task.

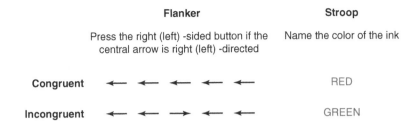

Fig. 1.10 Example of items from the flanker and Stroop tasks

Brain areas associated with the executive control system are the dorsal ACC and the dorsolateral PFC (Bush et al. 2000), although additional areas may be implicated when complex tasks are used (Fan et al. 2005). Thus, the ACC represents a possible anatomical locus of overlapping of executive control with vigilant attention (see Sect. 1.2 above). The ACC may also be important for error monitoring. For example, Carter et al. (1999) argued that this structure is involved in executive processes and that it serves an evaluative function in executive control, rather than a strictly strategic function. Functional MRI evidence with the attention network test (Fan et al. 2002) found ACC activation for the executive part of the task (Fan et al. 2005). Many studies revealed an involvement of the ACC in response conflict (e.g., in the Stroop task; Carter et al. 1995; Pardo 1990, or in verb generation; Barch et al. 2000). More generally, the ACC seems necessary to modify behavioral responses during challenging cognitive and physical states that require additional effortful cognitive control. Moreover, it monitors the emotional salience (pleasantness/aversiveness) of stimuli in relation with orbitofrontal cortex, exerts control over the autonomic nervous system with insular cortex, and modulates cognitive activity in conjunction with the dorsolateral PFC (Gasquoine 2013). Recent models (Silvetti et al. 2011; Brown 2013) stress a possible role for ACC in predicting and evaluating the outcome of planned actions, thus implementing the capacity of "thinking before acting", which is central to the concept of attentional control.

Some forms of inhibitory control on prepotent but inappropriate responses might also require the activity of ventrolateral PFC regions such as the inferior frontal gyrus, particularly in the right hemisphere (Aron et al. 2004; but see Hampshire et al. 2010).

References

Allport DA. Visual attention. In: Posner MI, editor. Foundations of cognitive science. Cambridge, MA: MIT Press; 1989. p. 631–87.

Anton-Erxleben K, Carrasco M. Attentional enhancement of spatial resolution: linking behavioural and neurophysiological evidence. Nat Rev Neurosci. 2013;14:188–200.

Aron AR, Robbins TW, Poldrack RA. Inhibition and the right inferior frontal cortex. Trends Cogn Sci. 2004;8:170–7.

Asplund CL, Todd JJ, Snyder AP, Marois R. A central role for the lateral prefrontal cortex in goal-directed and stimulus-driven attention. Nat Neurosci. 2010;13:507–12.

Aston-Jones G, Cohen JD. An integrative theory of locus coeruleus-norepinephrine function: adaptive gain and optimal performance. Annu Rev Neurosci. 2005;28:403–50.

Barch DM, Braver TS, Sabb FW, Noll DC. Anterior cingulate and the monitoring of response conflict: evidence from an fMRI study of overt verb generation. J Cogn Neurosci. 2000;12:298–309.

Bartolomeo P, Lupiáñez J, editors. Inhibitory after-effects in spatial processing: experimental and theoretical issues on inhibition of return. Hove: Psychology Press; 2006.

Bartolomeo P, Zieren N, Vohn R, Dubois B, Sturm W. Neural correlates of primary and reflective consciousness of spatial orienting. Neuropsychologia. 2008;46:348–61.

Bartolomeo P, Thiebaut de Schotten M, Chica AB. Brain networks of visuospatial attention and their disruption in visual neglect. Front Hum Neurosci. 2012;6:110.

Berlucchi G. Inhibition of return: a phenomenon in search of a mechanism and a better name. Cogn Neuropsychol. 2006;23:1065–74.

Bowers D, Heilman KM. Pseudoneglect: effects of hemispace on a tactile line bisection task. Neuropsychologia. 1980;18:491–8.

Brown JW. Beyond conflict monitoring: cognitive control and the neural basis of thinking before you act. Curr Dir Psychol Sci. 2013;22:179–85.

Buschman TJ, Miller EK. Top-down versus bottom-up control of attention in the prefrontal and posterior parietal cortices. Science. 2007;315:1860–2.

Bush G, Luu P, Posner MI. Cognitive and emotional influences in anterior cingulate cortex. Trends Cogn Sci. 2000;4:215–22.

Carrasco M, Ling S, Read S. Attention alters appearance. Nat Neurosci. 2004;7:308–13.

Carter CS, Mintun M, Cohen JD. Interference and facilitation effects during selective attention: an H215O PET study of Stroop task performance. Neuroimage. 1995;2:264–72.

Carter CS, Botvinick MM, Cohen JD. The contribution of the anterior cingulate cortex to executive processes in cognition. Rev Neurosci. 1999;10:49–57.

Catani M, Jones DK, Donato R, Ffytche DH. Occipito-temporal connections in the human brain. Brain. 2003;126:2093–107.

Chica AB, Bartolomeo P. Attentional routes to conscious perception. Front Psychol. 2012;3:1–12.

Chica AB, Bartolomeo P, Lupiáñez J. Two cognitive and neural systems for endogenous and exogenous spatial attention. Behav Brain Res. 2013a;237:107–23.

Chica AB, Paz-Alonso PM, Valero-Cabré A, Bartolomeo P. Neural bases of the interactions between spatial attention and conscious perception. Cereb Cortex. 2013b;23:1269–79.

Chun MM, Golomb JD, Turk-Browne NB. A taxonomy of external and internal attention. Annu Rev Psychol. 2011;62:73–101.

Corbetta M, Shulman GL. Control of goal-directed and stimulus-driven attention in the brain. Nat Rev Neurosci. 2002;3:201–15.

Coull JT, Buchel C, Friston KJ, Frith CD. Noradrenergically mediated plasticity in a human attentional neuronal network. Neuroimage. 1999;10:705–15.

Dehaene S, Changeux JP. Experimental and theoretical approaches to conscious processing. Neuron. 2011;70:200–27.

Desimone R, Duncan J. Neural mechanisms of selective visual attention. Annu Rev Neurosci. 1995;18:193–222.

Di Ferdinando A, Parisi D, Bartolomeo P. Modeling orienting behavior and its disorders with "ecological" neural networks. J Cogn Neurosci. 2007;19:1033–49.

Egly R, Driver J, Rafal RD. Shifting visual attention between objects and locations: evidence from normal and parietal lesion patients. J Exp Psychol Gen. 1994;123:161–77.

Eriksen BA, Eriksen CW. Effects of noise letters upon the identification of a target letter in a non-search task. Percept Psychophys. 1974;16:143–9.

Fan J, McCandliss BD, Sommer T, Raz A, Posner MI. Testing the efficiency and independence of attentional networks. J Cogn Neurosci. 2002;14:340–7.

Fan J, McCandliss BD, Fossella J, Flombaum JI, Posner MI. The activation of attentional networks. Neuroimage. 2005;26:471–9.

Fernandez-Duque D, Posner MI. Relating the mechanisms of orienting and alerting. Neuropsychologia. 1997;35:477–86.

Gaspar P, Berger B, Febvret A, Vigny A, Henry JP. Catecholamine innervation of the human cerebral cortex as revealed by comparative immunohistochemistry of tyrosine hydroxylase and dopamine-beta-hydroxylase. J Comp Neurol. 1989;279:249–71.

Gasquoine PG. Localization of function in anterior cingulate cortex: from psychosurgery to functional neuroimaging. Neurosci Biobehav Rev. 2013;37:340–8.

Gillebert CR, Mantini D, Peeters R, Dupont P, Vandenberghe R. Cytoarchitectonic mapping of attentional selection and reorienting in parietal cortex. Neuroimage. 2013;67:257–72.

Goodale MA, Milner AD. Separate visual pathways for perception and action. Trends Neurosci. 1992;15:20–5.

Hampshire A, Chamberlain SR, Monti MM, Duncan J, Owen AM. The role of the right inferior frontal gyrus: inhibition and attentional control. Neuroimage. 2010;50:1313–9.

Indovina I, Macaluso E. Dissociation of stimulus relevance and saliency factors during shifts of visuospatial attention. Cereb Cortex. 2007;17:1701–11.

Jewell G, McCourt ME. Pseudoneglect: a review and meta-analysis of performance factors in line bisection tasks. Neuropsychologia. 2000;38:93–110.

Klein RM. Inhibition of return. Trends Cogn Sci. 2000;4:138–47.

Kravitz DJ, Saleem KS, Baker CI, Mishkin M. A new neural framework for visuospatial processing. Nat Rev Neurosci. 2011;12:217–30.

Kravitz DJ, Saleem KS, Baker CI, Ungerleider LG, Mishkin M. The ventral visual pathway: an expanded neural framework for the processing of object quality. Trends Cogn Sci. 2013;17:26–49.

Kusnir F, Chica AB, Mitsumasu MA, Bartolomeo P. Phasic auditory alerting improves visual conscious perception. Conscious Cogn. 2011;20:1201–10.

LaBerge D, Auclair L, Siéroff E. Preparatory attention: experiment and theory. Conscious Cogn. 2000;9:396–434.

Lu C-H, Proctor RW. The influence of irrelevant location information on performance: a review of the Simon and spatial Stroop effects. Psychon Bull Rev. 1995;2:174–207.

Mack A, Rock I. Inattentional blindness. Cambridge, MA: The MIT Press; 1998.

Macquistan AD. Object-based allocation of visual attention in response to exogenous, but not endogenous, spatial precues. Psychon Bull Rev. 1997;4:512–5.

Maylor EA, Hockey R. Inhibitory component of externally controlled covert orienting in visual space. J Exp Psychol Hum Percept Perform. 1985;11:777–87.

Mesulam MM, Hersh LB, Mash DC, Geula C. Differential cholinergic innervation within functional subdivisions of the human cerebral cortex: a choline acetyltransferase study. J Comp Neurol. 1992;318:316–28.

Mishkin M, Ungerleider LG, Macko KA. Object vision and spatial vision: two cortical pathways. Trends Neurosci. 1983;6:414–7.

Moran J, Desimone R. Selective attention gates visual processing in the extrastriate cortex. Science. 1985;229:782–4.

Moruzzi G, Magoun HW. Brainstem reticular formation and activation of the EEG. Electroencephalogr Clin Neurophysiol. 1949;1:455–73.

Mottaghy FM, Willmes K, Horwitz B, Muller HW, Krause BJ, Sturm W. Systems level modeling of a neuronal network subserving intrinsic alertness. Neuroimage. 2006;29:225–33.

Parasuraman R. The attentive brain: issues and prospects. In: Parasuraman R, editor. The attentive brain. Cambridge, MA: The MIT Press; 1998. p. 3–15.

Pardo JV, Fox PT, Raichle ME. Localization of a human system for sustained attention by positron emission tomography. Nature. 1991;349:61–4.

Pardo JV, Pardo PJ, Janer KW, Raichle ME. The anterior cingulate cortex mediates processing selection in the Stroop attentional conflict paradigm. Proceedings of the National Academy of Sciences of the United States of America. 1990;87:256–9.

Paus T, Koski L, Caramanos Z, Westbury C. Regional differences in the effects of task difficulty and motor output on blood flow response in the human anterior cingulate cortex: a review of 107 PET activation studies. NeuroReport. 1998;9:R37–47.

Petrides M, Pandya DN. Projections to the frontal cortex from the posterior parietal region in the rhesus monkey. J Comp Neurol. 1984;228:105–16.

Posner MI. Orienting of attention. Q J Exp Psychol. 1980;32:3–25.

Posner MI. Attention: the mechanisms of consciousness. Proc Natl Acad Sci U S A. 1994;91:7398–403.

Posner MI, Cohen Y. Components of visual orienting. In: Bouma H, Bouwhuis D, editors. Attention and performance X. London: Lawrence Erlbaum; 1984. p. 531–56.

Posner MI, Rafal RD, Choate LS, Vaughan J. Inhibition of return: neural basis and function. Cogn Neuropsychol. 1985;2:211–28.

Rafal RD, Henik A. The neurology of inhibition: integrating controlled and automatic processes. In: Dagenbach D, Carr TH, editors. Inhibitory processes in attention, memory and language. San Diego: Academic; 1994. p. 1–51.

Rizzolatti G, Matelli M. Two different streams form the dorsal visual system: anatomy and functions. Exp Brain Res. 2003;153:146–57.

Robertson IH, Mattingley JB, Rorden C, Driver J. Phasic alerting of neglect patients overcomes their spatial deficit in visual awareness. Nature. 1998;395:169–72.

Robertson IH, Garavan H. Vigilant attention. In: Gazzaniga MS, editor. The cognitive neurosciences. 3rd ed. Cambridge, MA: MIT Press; 2004. p. 563–78.

Sadaghiani S, Scheeringa R, Lehongre K, Morillon B, Giraud AL, Kleinschmidt A. Intrinsic connectivity networks, alpha oscillations, and tonic alertness: a simultaneous electroencephalography/functional magnetic resonance imaging study. J Neurosci. 2010;30:10243–50.

Sarter M, Givens B, Bruno JP. The cognitive neuroscience of sustained attention: where top-down meets bottom-up. Behav Brain Res. 2001;35:146–60.

Schmahmann JD, Pandya DN. Fiber pathways of the brain. New York: Oxford University Press; 2006.

Silvetti M, Seurinck R, Verguts T. Value and prediction error in medial frontal cortex: integrating the single-unit and systems levels of analysis. Front Hum Neurosci. 2011;5:75.

Simons DJ, Chabris CF. Gorillas in our midst: sustained inattentional blindness for dynamic events. Perception. 1999;28:1059–74.

Singh-Curry V, Husain M. The functional role of the inferior parietal lobe in the dorsal and ventral stream dichotomy. Neuropsychologia. 2009;47:1434–48.

Stroop JR. Studies of interference in serial verbal reactions. J Exp Psychol. 1935;18:643–62.

Sturm W. Aufmerksamkeitsstörungen. In: Sturm W, Herrmann M, Münte TF, Hrsg. Lehrbuch der Klinischen Neuropsychologie. 2. Aufl. Heidelberg: Spektrum; 2009. p. 421–43.

Sturm W, Willmes K. On the functional neuroanatomy of intrinsic and phasic alertness. Neuroimage. 2001;14:S76–84.

Sturm W, de Simone A, Krause BJ, Specht K, Hesselmann V, Radermacher I, Herzog H, Tellmann L, Muller-Gartner HW, Willmes K. Functional anatomy of intrinsic alertness: evidence for a fronto-parietal-thalamic-brainstem network in the right hemisphere. Neuropsychologia. 1999;37:797–805.

Sturm W, Longoni F, Fimm B, Dietrich T, Weis S, Kemna S, Herzog H, Willmes K. Network for auditory intrinsic alertness: a PET study. Neuropsychologia. 2004;42:563–8.

Sundberg KA, Mitchell JF, Gawne TJ, Reynolds JH. Attention influences single unit and local field potential response latencies in visual cortical area v4. J Neurosci. 2012;32:16040–50.

Thiebaut de Schotten M, Dell'Acqua F, Forkel SJ, Simmons A, Vergani F, Murphy DGM, Catani M. A lateralized brain network for visuospatial attention. Nat Neurosci. 2011;14:1245–6.

Thiebaut de Schotten M, Cohen L, Amemiya E, Braga LW, Dehaene S. Learning to read improves the structure of the arcuate fasciculus. Cereb Cortex. 2012. doi:10.1093/cercor/bhs383 [Epub ahead of print].

Toba MN, Cavanagh P, Bartolomeo P. Attention biases the perceived midpoint of horizontal lines. Neuropsychologia 2011;49:238–346.

Wilkins AJ, Shallice T, McCarthy R. Frontal lesions and sustained attention. Neuropsychologia. 1987;25:359–65.

Wyart V, Tallon-Baudry C. Neural dissociation between visual awareness and spatial attention. J N eurosci. 2008;28:2667–79.

Yantis S. Attentional capture in vision. In: Kramer AF, Coles GH, Logan GD, editors. Converging operations in the study of visual selective attention. Washington, DC: American Psychological Association; 1995. p. 45–76.

Further Reading

Aston-Jones G, Cohen JD. An integrative theory of locus coeruleus-norepinephrine function: adaptive gain and optimal performance. Annu Rev Neurosci. 2005;28(1):403–50.

Bartolomeo P, Lupiáñez J, editors. Inhibitory after-effects in spatial processing: Experimental and theoretical issues on inhibition of return. Hove: Psychology Press; 2006.

Behrmann M, Geng JJ, Shomstein S. Parietal cortex and attention. Curr Opin Neurobiol. 2004;14(2):212–7.

Callejas A, Lupiáñez J, Funes MJ, Tudela P. Modulations among the alerting, orienting and executive control networks. Exp Brain Res. 2005;167(1):27–37.

Catani M, Thiebaut de Schotten M. Atlas of the human brain connections. Oxford: Oxford University Press; 2012.

Corbetta M, Shulman GL. Control of goal-directed and stimulus-driven attention in the brain. Nat Rev Neurosci. 2002;3(3):201–15.

Pashler HE. The psychology of attention. Cambridge, MA: MIT Press; 1998.

Petersen SE, Posner MI. The attention system of the human brain: 20 years after. Annu Rev Neurosci. 2012;35:73–89.

Robertson IH, Garavan H. Vigilant attention. In: Gazzaniga MS, editor. The cognitive neurosciences. 3rd ed. Cambridge, MA: MIT Press; 2004; p. 563–78.

Schmahmann JD, Pandya DN. Fiber pathways of the brain. New York: Oxford University Press; 2006.

Thiebaut de Schotten M, Dell'Acqua F, Forkel SJ, Simmons A, Vergani F, Murphy DGM, Catani M. A lateralized brain network for visuospatial attention. Nat Neurosci. 2011;14(10):1245–6.

Chapter 2
Sensorimotor Deficits After Right Brain Damage

Keywords Motor system • Visual processing • Somatosensory processing • Gaze position • Gaze deviation • Magnetic attraction of gaze

2.1 Hemiplegia, Hemianopia, and Hemianesthesia

The sensorimotor pathways are bilaterally organized across the hemispheres, so that each hemisphere mainly deals with the opposite side of space or the body.

The primary motor cortex is located in the anterior bank of the central sulcus. It connects to the motor neurons in the spinal cord, which innervate the skeletal muscles, through the corticospinal tract, which crosses the midline at the brain stem level. Damage to the motor cortex or to the corticospinal tract before its crossing typically provokes motor deficits of the contralateral limbs (hemiplegia). The somatosensory system originates in the sensory receptors in the skin, which connect with peripheral nerves. Peripheral nerves have their cell body in the dorsal root ganglia and enter the posterior columns of the spinal cord, terminating in the gracile and cuneate nuclei of the rostral cervical cord and medulla. From these nuclei, fibers cross the midline in the brain stem and ascend to terminate in the posterior thalamic nuclei. Thalamocortical connections reach the primary somatosensory cortex located in the postcentral gyrus, in the anterior portion of the parietal lobe, and a second somatosensory area in the upper bank of the lateral sulcus, adjacent to the insula. Injury of the posterior thalamus or of the cortical somatosensory areas results in contralateral disturbances of somatic sensation (hemianesthesia).

Figure 2.1 displays a schematic view of the visual pathways from the retina to the primary visual areas, as well as of the regions of visual loss after damage to different sites of the visual pathways. Visual signals processed by the retina travel along the optic nerve, which partially decussate at the level of the optic chiasm, so that each hemisphere receives information from the opposite visual field.

P. Bartolomeo, *Attention Disorders After Right Brain Damage*,
DOI 10.1007/978-1-4471-5649-9_2, © Springer-Verlag London 2014

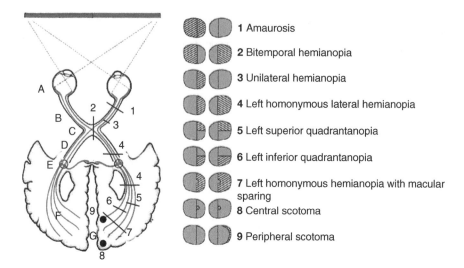

1 Amaurosis

2 Bitemporal hemianopia

3 Unilateral hemianopia

4 Left homonymous lateral hemianopia

5 Left superior quadrantanopia

6 Left inferior quadrantanopia

7 Left homonymous hemianopia with macular sparing

8 Central scotoma

9 Peripheral scotoma

Fig. 2.1 A schematic representation of the hemispheric organization of visual pathways and stations, with the deficits resulting from their lesion at different levels. *A* retina, *B* optic nerve, *C* optic chiasm, *D* optic tract, *E* lateral geniculate nucleus, *F* optic radiations, *G* primary visual cortex. Typically, disconnection of the lower part of the optic radiations, which runs in the temporal lobe, gives rise to loss of vision in the superior quadrants of the opposite hemifield (superior quadrantanopia); lesion of the dorsal components of the optic radiations in the depth of the parietal lobe determines inferior quadrantanopia (Modified from Bartolomeo and Migliaccio (2011). © 2011, with permission from Il Mulino)

The optic tracts make a synaptic stop in the lateral geniculate nucleus, the thalamic station of the visual system. Caudally to the geniculate, the optic radiations expand in the white matter of the temporal and parietal lobes to reach the primary visual cortex (BA 17) in the occipital lobe. Damage at each stage of these pathways can provoke loss of vision in different sectors of the visual fields (see Fig. 2.1). Unilateral lesions posterior to the geniculate nucleus, affecting the optic radiations or the primary visual cortex, often induce visual loss in the contralateral halves or quarters of the visual fields, called lateral homonymous hemianopia or quadrantanopia.

Visual fields can be tested clinically by the confrontation method. The examiner is in front of the patient and outstretches his/her hands in the patient's visual field. The patient fixates the examiner's nose and reports the movement of the examiner's fingers in his/her visual fields. A more accurate test is perimetry. The patient is in front of a hollow white spherical bowl (Goldmann perimeter), with one eye covered. The patient fixates a central point and is asked to detect a test light of variable size and intensity presented by the examiner in the patient's visual periphery. The procedure is now often automatic, with the patient pressing a button when he/she perceives the stimulus light.

As a consequence of the anatomical organization of the sensory and motor pathways, brain lesions affecting these systems should provoke (mostly) contralateral deficits with equal prevalence after right or left hemisphere damage. However, when Meador et al. (1988) assessed tactile perception in 18 patients undergoing preoperative evaluation for epilepsy surgery by injecting sodium Amytal into one carotid artery, which selectively inactivates the ipsilateral hemisphere, they observed a greater frequency of tactile deficits (lack of detection or extinction of contralateral stimuli, see Sect. 2.2 below) during right injections than during left injections. Sterzi et al. (1993) assessed sensorimotor functions in a continuous series of 154 left-brain-damaged and 144 right-brain-damaged stroke patients. They found that visual half-field and motor deficits, as well as disorders of position sense, were more frequent in right-brain-damaged than in left-brain-damaged patients. A similar tendency occurred for deficits of pain sensation. This result might in part be influenced by a recruitment bias. Patients with relatively minor left hemisphere lesions and language disorders may be more likely to seek medical help than patients with equivalent right hemisphere damage, who might not notice their deficits. Anosognosia in right-brain-damaged patients (see Sect. 3.2) may also contribute to their failure to acknowledge their deficits. As a result, when lesion volume is not assessed, right-brain-damaged patients might have generally larger lesions than left-brain-damaged patients. There is, however, the alternative possibility that cognitive deficits specific to right hemisphere lesions simulated sensorimotor deficits, consistent with the results by Meador et al. (1988). In agreement with this hypothesis, a patient with an ischemic lesion of the right occipital and temporal lobes showed clinical signs of left homonymous hemianopia, which however greatly improved when his gaze was deviated 30° to the right, so that the left retinotopic field was in his right hemispace (Nadeau and Heilman 1991). Another patient with apparent hemianopia on standard perimetry and signs of visual neglect after a right parietal lesion (see Chap. 4) became able to report left-sided stimuli when the fixation point was removed prior to stimulus onset, thus decreasing the competition between the left-sided stimulus and the fixation point situated to its right (Walker et al. 1991).

These cases of *pseudo-hemianopia* indicate that, in patients with right hemisphere damage, traditional testing for visual field defects can lead to incorrect diagnosis, because patients' behavioral responses may be influenced by attention deficits. Objective techniques such as evoked potentials are better suited to discriminate between sensory and cognitive problems. Indeed, Vallar et al. (1991) recorded somatosensory or visual evoked potentials for stimuli contralateral and ipsilateral to the lesion in three patients with right hemisphere lesions and signs of left neglect and in three patients with left brain damage and no neglect. All patients had contralateral homonymous hemianopia or hemianesthesia. The three neglect patients showed normal evoked potentials for left-sided stimuli, despite the absence of conscious perception or verbal report of the stimuli. In contrast, the three left-brain-damaged patients without neglect showed no detectable cortical evoked response to contralateral visual or somatosensory stimuli. Vallar et al. (1991) concluded that in patients with visual neglect, hemianopia and hemianesthesia may be manifestations of neglect, rather than representing primary sensory deficit. This hypothesis can account for the greater frequency of (apparent) sensory deficits after right hemisphere lesions than after left brain damage. Attention processes might well be the functional locus of impairment in these patients. A functional MRI study (Vuilleumier et al. 2008) demonstrated preserved BOLD responses to left-sided stimuli in the right visual cortex in patients with right parietal lesions and left neglect. However, responses to the same stimuli were pathologically reduced when attentional load at fixation was increased. Thus, disorders resulting from damage to attention networks can impair the functioning of anatomically intact primary sensory areas.

2.2 Perceptual Extinction

Perceptual extinction was originally described by Loeb (1885) and Oppenheim (1885). The extinction phenomenon refers to a dissociation in patients' performance between normal detection of a stimulus presented alone on the side contralateral to a hemispheric lesion and lack of report of that same stimulus when another stimulus is presented simultaneously on the side ipsilateral to the lesion. In other words, it is as if the contralesional stimulus could be normally processed when presented in isolation, but under bilateral simultaneous stimulation, it would systematically lose the competition with the ipsilesional stimulus and thus be "extinguished" by it. This disorder was called *extinction* by Bender (1952) or *sensory inattention* by Critchley (1953).

Extinction can occur for stimuli presented in various sensory modalities: visual (Vuilleumier and Rafal 2000), somatosensory (Bartolomeo et al. 2004), acoustic (De Renzi et al. 1984), olfactory (Bellas et al. 1988), and even cross modally (Mattingley et al. 1997).

Somatosensory extinction can be tested by asking the blindfolded patient to report when the examiner lightly touches the patient's limbs or face. Interestingly, the spatial position of the limbs has been shown to influence extinction rates, thus indicating that tactile extinction does not depend solely on sensory factors. Crossing of hands, so that each hand is on the opposite side of the body midline relative to the other, was shown to improve detection of stimuli given to the left hand by 30 % (Aglioti et al. 1999). In another study, however, where patients were requested to cross both arms and legs (Bartolomeo et al. 2004), limb crossing induced a deterioration of performance for stimuli applied to right body parts, with only a tendency to an improvement of detection for left body parts. Thus, in conditions of high attentional load, limb crossing may impair tactile detection in most patients with left extinction and particularly in those showing signs of left visual neglect. These results underline the importance of general attentional capacity in the determination of tactile extinction.

To examine auditory (or acoustic) extinction, the examiner may lightly snap his/her fingers and make a clicking sound near the patients' ears. Patients may not report the contralesional noise on bilateral presentation. In the auditory domain, it is difficult to discriminate between extinction and auditory neglect (Gokhale et al. 2013) (see Chaps. 4, 5, and 6).

2.2.1 Allesthesia

During clinical examination, *allesthesia*, another phenomenon typical of right hemisphere damage, may occur. In allesthesia, a contralesional (usually left-sided) stimulus is reported as occurring at an ipsilesional (usually right-sided), unstimulated location. This comparatively rare spatial disorder of stimulus localization is typically observed in the somatosensory, visual, or acoustic modality, but, like extinction, it can occur between different modalities, such as touch and audition. For example, an 84-year-old patient with an ischemic right frontoparietal lesion, who showed moderate signs of left extrapersonal neglect and left extinction in the visual, acoustic, and tactile modalities, as well as between modalities, spontaneously reported left-sided acoustic stimuli as occurring at her right-sided ear or hand (Ortigue et al. 2005). Even more rarely, the opposite phenomenon may occur in anesthesia of central origin, perhaps without any preferential laterality of brain lesion. In 6 patients with hands rendered anesthetic by unilateral hemispheric lesions of vascular or neurosurgical origins, firm pressure on the healthy hand was sometimes perceived on the other, anesthetized hand (Sathian 2000), similar to phantom limb amputee patients who may refer a touch on their normal hand to their phantom limb (Ramachandran et al. 1995).

2.2.2 Mechanisms of Extinction

Extinction and unilateral neglect (see Chaps. 4, 5, 6, and 7) are often associated phenomena, because the phenomenon of extinction (and particularly visual extinction) is often observed even in mild forms of neglect or as a sequel of neglect. Indeed, extinction often persists as a residual symptom after recovery from neglect (Robertson and Halligan 1999). These similarities could suggest similar underlying deficits, such as attention deficits (Posner et al. 1984; Kinsbourne 1987). However, a certain degree of independence between the two phenomena seems to exist, since even peripheral lesions can lead to extinction (Heilman et al. 1993). Extinction and neglect can also dissociate, both from a clinical perspective (Cocchini et al. 1999) and in terms of lesion localization (Bisiach et al. 1989; Vallar et al. 1994). However, it is worth noting that, similar to what happens in neglect, the probability of a stimulus being neglected does not only depends on its absolute location in space (e.g., right or left visual field) but also on the spatial relationships it has with the "extinguisher" stimulus. Even within a single hemifield, a stimulus can go unreported if it is presented on the left-hand side relative to the extinguished stimulus (Kinsbourne 1977). For example, a patient with left visual extinction reported by Di Pellegrino and De Renzi (1995) extinguished the leftmost of two stimuli presented in the left hemispace, while he always perceived both stimuli when they were presented in the right space. However, when asked to purposefully ignore the right-sided stimulus, left extinctions decreased.

Accounts of extinction typically emphasize either a sensory problem not severe enough to impair perception of single stimuli (Bender 1952) or an attentional disorder favoring ipsilateral over contralateral stimuli (Critchley 1953), or both (Marzi et al. 2001). Attentional deficits in visual extinction were explored by Baylis et al. (1993), who asked five patients with visual extinction following unilateral brain damage to locate and report the color and the shape of letters presented in either or both visual fields. On double simultaneous stimulation, patients tended to extinguish the event contralateral to their lesion and then especially when the two stimuli were the same in the reported dimension (either color or shape). The authors concluded that the visual system can normally process extinguished colors and shapes up to a certain extent, even though they are unavailable for verbal report. One possibility is that extinction might reflect an inability for the contralesional stimulus to access a decision center located in the left hemisphere (Marzi et al. 2001). If so, then the use of nonverbal responses should decrease left extinction by rendering less important the left hemisphere contribution to response. This was indeed the case for one patient with right frontoparietal damage (Smania et al. 1996). This patient had a high rate of left misses on bilateral visual stimulation when responding verbally or when using his right hand. However, left extinction decreased dramatically when he was asked to respond by lowering the chin or by moving his eyes. These nonverbal responses are based on bilateral muscle activity, which is organized across both hemispheres.

The attention deficits in extinction might reflect an impaired token-individuation process (Vuilleumier 2013), whereby a stimulus cannot be identified as a particular object occurring in a specific time and location (see Kahneman et al. 1992). The right IPL might play an important role in this process, perhaps by integrating activity in dorsal and ventral cortical visual pathways (Vuilleumier 2013), respectively dedicated to spatial attention and perceptual processes (see Sect. 1.1.4). Consistent with this proposal, Vuilleumier and Rafal (2000) described patients with visual extinction who could enumerate the very same multiple simultaneous stimuli they were unable to report. In this case, it was hypothesized that enumeration would not call for attending to individual stimuli, but for abilities requiring less attention, such as subitizing (i.e., the capacity to judge the number of small sets of objects without counting).

2.2.3 Attention and Extinction

There is a possible pathophysiological kinship between extinction and neglect (see Chaps. 4, 5, 6, and 7), based on the fact that a component of magnetic attraction of attention to the stimulus located ipsilateral to the lesion may contribute to the phenomenon of extinction (Gainotti et al. 2008). A critical component of the phenomenon of magnetic attraction is indeed the presentation of a distractor-extinguisher stimulus on the side ipsilateral to the brain lesion. Consistent with these notions, the exploration of the electrophysiological correlates of left visual extinction in a patient with right hemisphere damage demonstrated a selective absence of the early attention-sensitive P1 (80–120 ms) and N1 (140–180 ms) components of the ERP for extinguished stimuli (Marzi et al. 2000).

Also, damage to attention-related PPC sites has been stressed as a lesional correlate of visual extinction. In particular, TPJ often seems to be lesioned in these patients (Karnath et al. 2003; Molenberghs et al. 2012). Using the Posner RT paradigm (see Chap. 1), Friedrich et al. (1998) demonstrated the presence of a pattern of RT resembling extinction in patients with TPJ damage, but not in patients with more dorsal lesions in the SPL. This pattern corresponds to the disengagement deficit (see Sect. 6.1), i.e., disproportionally slowed RTs for left-sided targets preceded by right-sided cues. An anatomical and neuroimaging study (Gillebert et al. 2011) on patients with parietal damage, including two patients with left and right parietal damages, respectively, indicated instead a role for IPS damage without involvement of more ventral sites such as TPJ. However, in the case of IPS damage, contralesional extinction was equally present after right or left hemisphere lesions.

A critical role of attention deficits in extinction is also confirmed by functional MRI studies that compared brain responses to the same contralesional stimuli when they were presented unilaterally and correctly perceived or with a concomitant ipsilesional stimulus and, consequently, missed. These studies consistently revealed preserved activation of primary sensory areas for extinguished stimuli in the visual modality (Vuilleumier et al. 2001), as well as in the somatosensory modality (Beversdorf et al. 2008).

2.3   Motor Neglect

In his seminal book *The Parietal Lobes,* Macdonald Critchley (1953) listed the chief clinical features which suggest that the parietal lobe be affected in a case of hemiparesis (Critchley 1953). The first item he mentioned is "greater poverty of movement than can be accounted for on the basis of paralysis." A decrease of spontaneous motor activity which cannot be explained by direct damage to the motor system has long been recognized and dubbed *motor neglect* by Laplane and Degos (1983).

At variance with directional motor disorders such as directional hypokinesia (see Sect. 4.4.2), where the impairment concerns left-directed movements independent of the effector used, in motor neglect patients are reluctant to use their left limbs, independent of the sector of extrapersonal space where the movement should be executed (left or right). Importantly, motor neglect does not depend on deficits of muscle strength. In its pure form, which is rare, the patient acts as if he or she were hemiplegic; however, with a strong incentive, he/she can mobilize the contralesional limbs with a force close to normal. In the original description (Laplane and Degos 1983), slowing of gestures and loss of placement reactions and of avoidance responses to noxious stimuli were also mentioned. Motor neglect can be observed in the absence of spatial neglect (Barbieri and De Renzi 1989). The phenomenon of motor neglect seems similar to *motor extinction*, characterized by akinesia which occurs only when the subject must make a simultaneous movement of both hands (Valenstein and Heilman 1981).

Motor neglect refers to the behavior of brain-damaged patients who seem unwilling to initiate movements with the limbs contralateral to their brain lesion. Motor neglect is characterized by the loss of spontaneous utilization of a limb on one side, in the absence of deficits of strength, reflexes, or sensibility. The functional and lesional relationships with visual neglect are currently uncertain. Motor neglect has a clear clinical relevance, because patients can behave as if they were hemiplegic without having a primary motor deficit. For example, patients with motor neglect can either stumble upon their neglected foot or sit on their hand.

An early case of motor neglect was reported by Garcin et al. (1938). As a consequence of a glioblastoma in the right temporoparietal region, this patient showed a marked deficit of motor initiative in his left leg and arm in the absence of elementary motor deficits. There was a deficit of deep sensitivity with normal superficial sensitivity. Despite the absence of elementary motor deficits, he could not stand without help, because his left leg tended to give way. When reclining in bed, he forgot to lift his left leg. He also mistakenly considered as his own left hand the hand of another person put in front of him. The only thing which astonished him was that the stranger's hand could move, because he considered his left hand as paralyzed.

2.4 Conjugate Gaze Paresis

In the acute phase, patients with large strokes in the right hemisphere often lie in bed with their head and eyes turned towards the right side. It is often said that these patients "look at their brain lesions." This tonic gaze deviation is also known as Prévost's or Vulpian's sign (Larner 2010). Patients typically do not answer if questioned from the left side and cannot pay attention to the left even if summoned to do so. The tendency to rightward orienting is so compulsive and pervasive in this stage that it is usually impossible to administer neuropsychological tests.

In neurology textbooks, conjugate gaze paresis towards the lesioned hemisphere is often considered as symmetrically resulting from lesions be they to the left or the right FEF. However, a systematic study by De Renzi et al. (1982) on 436 consecutive patients with unilateral brain damage challenged this view. They found gaze paresis in 120 patients with more severe neurological impairment and higher mortality. However, contrary to the received wisdom, conjugate gaze paresis was also dependent on the side and locus of the lesion. It was more frequent, severe, and long-lasting in patients with right-sided brain damage. Moreover, it was predominantly associated with post-Rolandic lesions in patients with right-sided brain damage and with involvement of the entire territory of distribution of the middle cerebral artery in those with left-sided brain damage. Also, all the right-brain-damaged patients who had signs of gaze paresis at the time of examination also showed signs of left neglect (see Chap. 4). In addition, there were 15 patients who no longer showed gaze paresis yet, nevertheless, manifested neglect. The authors also observed the presence of marked gaze paresis in comatose patients. Thus, conjugate gaze paresis appears to be a consequence of damage in post-Rolandic regions of the right hemisphere and is often associated with disorders bearing a strong attentional component, such as visuospatial neglect (see Chap. 4).

2.5   "Magnetic" Gaze Attraction

After a few days, stroke patients usually recover the ability to maintain the head and eyes straight. However, the mere appearance of any visual object either on the right side or bilaterally can then induce an immediate orientation of the patient's head and eyes towards the right-sided object. For example, in testing the visual fields by means of the confrontation technique, as soon as the examiner outstretches his or her hands, patients may look at the hand on their right, before the actual administration of the stimuli ("magnetic attraction" of gaze, Gainotti et al. 1991). Ipsilateral automatic capture of gaze, originally described by Fisher (1956) and referred to as "magnetic attraction of the gaze" by Cohn (1972), consists in the tendency to spontaneously orient gaze to the right as soon as the examiner raises his/her hands in the patients' visual fields and even before the examiner moves his/her fingers to stimulate the patient's attention. The tonic deviation of the head and eyes to the side opposite the hemiplegia and the automatic capture of gaze to stimuli appearing on the side ipsilateral to the lesion are observed more often after right brain injury than after left lesions and are closely associated with severe forms of neglect (De Renzi et al. 1982; Gainotti et al. 1991). Friedland and Weinstein (1977) considered magnetic attraction as an oculomotor analogue of visual extinction. Healthy subjects can behave in a similar way when their gaze is unwillingly attracted by the sudden onset of an irrelevant peripheral stimulus; they can make a saccade towards the distractor without knowing it (Theeuwes et al. 1998), an occurrence sometimes referred to as a "visual grasp reflex."

2.6   Conclusion: Apparent Sensorimotor Deficits After Right Hemisphere Damage

In some patients, right hemisphere lesions can induce apparent sensorimotor deficits. These include pseudo-hemianopia (Kooistra and Heilman 1989), whereby patients fail to acknowledge the presence of isolated left-sided stimuli (even in the absence of a competing right-sided stimulus); an apparent hemianesthesia (Vallar et al. 1991), with impaired perception of isolated left-sided tactile stimuli; or, as described in Sect. 2.3, a "cognitive" form of hemiplegia such as motor neglect. Bodily related deficits that can occur after right brain damage are resumed in Table 2.1. Thus, before concluding for an apparently elementary sensory or motor deficit, the clinician must keep in mind that such deficits can in fact result from higher-order impairments, especially after lesions of the right hemisphere.

Table 2.1 Bodily related cognitive deficits related to hemispheric damage, in approximate order of clinical importance (see Chap. 3)

Condition	Characteristics	Associated lesions
Anosognosia	Unawareness of disease (typically of left hemiplegia). It can take the minor form of anosodiaphoria or lack of concern for disease	Right insula and adjacent subcortical structures, premotor cortex, dorsal ACC, TPJ and medial temporal structures (hippocampus and amygdala)
Motor neglect	Unwillingness to initiate movements with the limbs contralateral to a brain lesion	Uncertain; supplementary and pre-supplementary motor areas?
Asomatognosia	Denial of ownership of left limbs, sometimes accompanied by delusional aspects (somatoparaphrenia)	Extensive fronto–temproroparietal lesions in the right hemisphere. Supramarginal gyrus of the IPL and underlying white matter. Insula, basal ganglia, thalamus, subcortical white matter, or in the territory of the anterior cerebral artery (cingulate gyrus, supplementary motor area, genu of the corpus callosum)
Misoplegia	Dislike, aversion and hostility towards the left side of the body	Right parietal lobe
Xenomelia	Feeling of disownership of a limb, which is asked to be amputated	No acquired brain damage; signs of decreased cortical thickness or surface in the SPL, somatosensory cortices, IPL, and anterior insula
Supernumerary phantom limbs	Feeling of the presence of one or more supernumerary limbs	Large right hemisphere lesions including TPJ and basal ganglia
Autoscopic hallucinations	Patients falsely perceive an image of their own body without identifying themselves with the hallucinated body	Extrastriate visual cortex, most often in the right hemisphere
Out-of-body experiences	Seeing a second own body from an elevated perspective	Right TPJ
Heautoscopy	Self-identification with a second own body, duplication of the subject's experience of the world	Temporal lobe, insula in the left hemisphere
Acute hemiconcern	Exceedingly caring attitude towards the left limbs, with relentless exploration and manipulation, during the first days after a right hemisphere stroke	Postcentral gyrus, superior and middle temporal gyri, anterior part of inferior parietal gyrus, and supramarginal gyrus of the right hemisphere

References

Aglioti S, Smania N, Peru A. Frames of reference for mapping tactile stimuli in brain-damaged patients. J Cogn Neurosci. 1999;11:67–79.

Barbieri C, De Renzi E. Patterns of neglect dissociation. Behav Neurol. 1989;2:13–4.

Bartolomeo P, Migliaccio R. I disturbi del riconoscimento: le agnosie. In: Vallar G, Papagno C, editors. Manuale di neuropsicologia clinica ed elementi di riabilitazione. 2nd ed. Bologna: Il Mulino; 2011.

Bartolomeo P, Perri R, Gainotti G. The influence of limb crossing on left tactile extinction. J Neurol Neurosurg Psychiatry. 2004;75:49–55.

Baylis GC, Driver J, Rafal RD. Visual extinction and stimulus repetition. J Cogn Neurosci. 1993;5:453–66.

Bellas DN, Novelly RA, Eskenazi B, Wasserstein J. The nature of unilateral neglect in the olfactory sensory system. Neuropsychologia. 1988;26:45–52.

Bender MB. Disorders in perception. Springfield: Thomas; 1952.

Beversdorf DQ, Hughes JD, Heilman KM. Functional MRI of the primary somatosensory cortex in extinction to simultaneous bilateral tactile stimuli due to right temporal lobe stroke. Neurocase. 2008;14:419–24.

Bisiach E, Vallar G, Geminiani G. Influence of response modality on perceptual awareness of contralesional visual stimuli. Brain. 1989;112(Pt 6):1627–36.

Cocchini G, Cubelli R, Della Sala S, Beschin N. Neglect without extinction. Cortex. 1999;35:285–313.

Cohn R. Eyeball movements in homonymous hemianopia following simultaneous bitemporal object presentation. Neurology. 1972;22:12–4.

Critchley M. The parietal lobes. New York: Hafner; 1953.

De Renzi E, Colombo A, Faglioni P, Gibertoni M. Conjugate gaze paresis in stroke patients with unilateral damage: an unexpected instance of hemispheric asymmetry. Arch Neurol. 1982;39:482–6.

De Renzi E, Gentilini M, Pattacini F. Auditory extinction following hemisphere damage. Neuropsychologia. 1984;22:733–44.

Di Pellegrino G, De Renzi E. An experimental investigation on the nature of extinction. Neuropsychologia. 1995;33:153–70.

Fisher M. Left hemiplegia and motor impersistence. J Nerv Ment Dis. 1956;123:201–18.

Friedland RP, Weinstein EA. Hemi-inattention and hemisphere specialization: introduction and historical review. In: Weinstein EA, Friedland RP, editors. Hemi-inattention and hemisphere specialization. New York: Raven Press; 1977.

Friedrich FJ, Egly R, Rafal RD, Beck D. Spatial attention deficits in humans: a comparison of superior parietal and temporal-parietal junction lesions. Neuropsychology. 1998;12:193–207.

Gainotti G, D'Erme P, Bartolomeo P. Early orientation of attention toward the half space ipsilateral to the lesion in patients with unilateral brain damage. J Neurol Neurosurg Psychiatry. 1991;54:1082–9.

Gainotti G, Bourlon C, Bartolomeo P. La négligence spatiale unilatérale. In: Lechevalier B, Viader F, Eustache F, editors. Traité de neuropsychologie clinique. Bruxelles/Paris: De Boeck/INSERM; 2008. p. 627–49.

Garcin R, Varay A, Hadji-Dimo. Document pour servir à l'étude des troubles du schéma corporel (sur quelques phénomènes moteurs, gnosiques et quelques troubles de l'utilisation des membres du côté gauche au cours d'un syndrome temporo-pariétal par tumeur, envisagés dans leurs rapports avec l'anosognosie et les troubles du schéma corporel). Revue Neurologique (Paris). 1938;69:498–510.

Gillebert CR, Mantini D, Thijs V, Sunaert S, Dupont P, Vandenberghe R. Lesion evidence for the critical role of the intraparietal sulcus in spatial attention. Brain. 2011;134:1694–709.

Gokhale S, Lahoti S, Caplan LR. The neglected neglect: auditory neglect. JAMA Neurol. 2013;70:1065–9.

Heilman KM, Watson RT, Valenstein E. Neglect and related disorders. In: Heilman KM, Valenstein E, editors. Clinical neuropsychology. 3rd ed. New York: Oxford University Press; 1993. p. 279–336.

Kahneman D, Treisman A, Gibbs BJ. The reviewing of object files: object-specific integration of information. Cogn Psychol. 1992;24:175–219.

Karnath H-O, Himmelbach M, Kuker W. The cortical substrate of visual extinction. NeuroReport. 2003;14:437–42.

Kinsbourne M. Hemi-neglect and hemisphere rivalry. In: Weinstein EA, Friedland RP, editors. Hemi-inattention and hemisphere specialization. New York: Raven Press; 1977. p. 41–9.

Kinsbourne M. Mechanisms of unilateral neglect. In: Jeannerod M, editor. Neurophysiological and neuropsychological aspects of spatial neglect. Amsterdam: Elsevier Science Publishers; 1987. p. 69–86.

Kooistra CA, Heilman KM. Hemispatial visual inattention masquerading as hemianopia. Neurology. 1989;39:1125–7.

Laplane D, Degos JD. Motor neglect. J Neurol Neurosurg Psychiatry. 1983;46:152–8.

Larner AJ. A dictionary of neurological signs. 3rd ed. New York: Springer; 2010.

Loeb J. Die elementaren Stoerungen einfacher Functionen nach oberflachlicher umschriebener Verletzung des Grosshirns Plugers. Arch Physiol. 1885;37:51–6.

Marzi CA, Girelli M, Miniussi C, Smania N, Maravita A. Electrophysiological correlates of conscious vision: evidence from unilateral extinction. J Cogn Neurosci. 2000;12:869–77.

Marzi CA, Girelli M, Natale E, Miniussi C. What exactly is extinguished in unilateral visual extinction? Neurophysiological evidence. Neuropsychologia. 2001;39:1354–66.

Mattingley JB, Driver J, Beschin N, Robertson IH. Attentional competition between modalities: extinction between touch and vision after right hemisphere damage. Neuropsychologia. 1997;35:867–80.

Meador KJ, Loring DW, Lee GP, Brooks BS, Thompson EE, Thompson WO, Heilman KM. Right cerebral specialization for tactile attention as evidenced by intracarotid sodium amytal. Neurology. 1988;38:1763–6.

Molenberghs P, Sale MV, Mattingley JB. Is there a critical lesion site for unilateral spatial neglect? A meta-analysis using activation likelihood estimation. Front Hum Neurosci. 2012;6:78.

Nadeau SE, Heilman KM. Gaze-dependent hemianopia without hemispatial neglect. Neurology. 1991;41:1244–50.

Oppenheim H. Ueber eine durch eine klinische bisher nich verwertete Untersuschungmethode ermittelte Form der Sensibitatsstoerung bei einsetigen Erkrankunger des Grosshirns. Neurologische Zentralblatt. 1885;4:529–33.

Ortigue S, Jabaudon D, Landis T, Michel CM, Maravita A, Blanke O. Preattentive interference between touch and audition: a case study on multisensory alloesthesia. NeuroReport. 2005;16:865–8.

Posner MI, Walker JA, Friedrich FJ, Rafal RD. Effects of parietal injury on covert orienting of attention. J Neurosci. 1984;4:1863–74.

Ramachandran VS, Rogers-Ramachandran D, Cobb S. Touching the phantom limb. Nature. 1995;377:489–90.

Robertson IH, Halligan P. Spatial neglect: a clinical handbook for diagnosis and treatment. Hove: Psychology Press; 1999.

Sathian KMP. Intermanual referral of sensation to anesthetic hands. Neurology. 2000;54:1866–8.

Smania N, Martini MC, Prior M, Marzi CA. Input and response determinants of visual extinction: a case study. Cortex. 1996;32:567–91.

Sterzi R, Bottini G, Celani MG, Righetti E, Lamassa M, Ricci S, Vallar G. Hemianopia, hemian-aesthesia, and hemiplegia after right and left hemisphere damage. A hemispheric difference. J Neurol Neurosurg Psychiatry. 1993;56:308–10.

Theeuwes J, Kramer AF, Hahn S, Irwin DE. Our eyes do not always go where we want them to go: capture of the eyes by new objects. Psychol Sci. 1998;9:379–85.

Valenstein E, Heilman KM. Unilateral hypokinesia and motor extinction. Neurology. 1981;31:445–8.

Vallar G, Sandroni P, Rusconi ML, Barbieri S. Hemianopia, hemianesthesia, and spatial neglect: a study with evoked potentials. Neurology. 1991;41:1918–22.

Vallar G, Rusconi ML, Bignamini L, Geminiani G, Perani D. Anatomical correlates of visual and tactile extinction in humans: a clinical CT scan correlation study in man. J Neurol Neurosurg Psychiatry. 1994;57:464–70.

Vuilleumier P. Mapping the functional neuroanatomy of spatial neglect and human parietal lobe functions: progress and challenge. Ann NY Acad Sci. 2013;1296(1):50–74.

Vuilleumier PO, Rafal RD. A systematic study of visual extinction. Between- and within-field deficits of attention in hemispatial neglect. Brain. 2000;123(Pt 6):1263–79.

Vuilleumier P, Sagiv N, Hazeltine E, Poldrack RA, Swick D, Rafal RD, Gabrieli JD. Neural fate of seen and unseen faces in visuospatial neglect: a combined event-related functional MRI and event-related potential study. Proc Natl Acad Sci U S A. 2001;98:3495–500.

Vuilleumier P, Schwartz S, Verdon V, Maravita A, Hutton C, Husain M, Driver J. Abnormal attentional modulation of retinotopic cortex in parietal patients with spatial neglect. Curr Biol. 2008;18:1525–9.

Walker R, Findlay JM, Young AW, Welch J. Disentangling neglect and hemianopia. Neuropsychologia. 1991;29:1019–27.

Further Reading

Bender MB. Disorders in perception. Springfield: Thomas; 1952.

Brozzoli C, Dematte ML, Pavani F, Frassinetti F, Farné A. Neglect and extinction: within and between sensory modalities. Restor Neurol Neurosci. 2006;24:217–32.

Driver J, Mattingley JB, Rorden C, Davis G. Extinction as a paradigm measure of attentional bias and restricted capacity following brain injury. In: Thier P, Karnath HO, editors. Parietal lobe contributions to orientation in 3D-space. Heidelberg: Springer; 1997. p. 401–29.

Vuilleumier P. Mapping the functional neuroanatomy of spatial neglect and human parietal lobe functions: progress and challenge. Ann NY Acad Sci. 2013;1296(1):50–74.

Chapter 3
Consequences of Right Hemisphere Lesions on Bodily Awareness and Control

Keywords Perceptual awareness • Motor control • Agency • Ownership • Awareness • Emotion • Body parts

3.1 Body-Related Cognition in the Right Hemisphere

In the large majority of right-handed individuals, as well as in many left-handed ones, the left hemisphere is dominant for several aspects of language abilities (Hervé et al. 2013). As a consequence, until a few decades ago, the right hemisphere was traditionally considered to be the "minor" hemisphere. However, we know now that the right hemisphere has essential functions, for example, in the domain of attention processes (see Chap. 1).

Importantly, some clinical consequences of brain lesions are relatively characteristic of right hemisphere damage. Although some of these conditions can also occur after left hemisphere damage, such cases occur much less frequently. Central among right hemisphere, neurological conditions are disorders of awareness, emotional reaction, ownership, agency, or control with respect to a patient's own body.

As a first example we consider delusional misidentifications, often observed after right hemisphere damage. Such damage may produce delusional verbalizations concerning a patient's left limbs, which may no longer be perceived as belonging to the patient's self, such is the case with *asomatognosia* and *somatoparaphrenia* (Gerstmann 1942; Critchley 1953). Delusional misidentifications of other persons' identity, such as the Capgras and Fregoli syndromes, are also sometimes associated with lesions in the right hemisphere, particularly in the frontal lobe (Feinberg and Keenan 2005). Also the delusional belief of being in another place, so-called reduplicative paramnesia, has been associated with frontal damage in the right hemisphere (Lee et al. 2011).

Such consequences of right hemisphere damage may blur the ego boundaries, impair self-monitoring, and produce inappropriate emotional reactions to external stimuli such as erroneous familiarity or feelings of estrangement (Devinsky 2009),

P. Bartolomeo, *Attention Disorders After Right Brain Damage*,
DOI 10.1007/978-1-4471-5649-9_3, © Springer-Verlag London 2014

thus perhaps disrupting the feelings of "warmth and intimacy and immediacy" (James 1890, p. 239) and the "resemblance among the parts of a continuum of feelings (especially bodily feelings)" (James 1890, p. 336), which are the foundation of personal identity according to William James. On the other hand, a left hemisphere receiving inadequate input from the damaged right hemisphere may produce "positive" symptoms such as delusional, confabulatory narratives (Devinsky 2009).

Thus, the functioning of the right hemisphere, and perhaps especially of fronto-parietal networks associated with attention processes (see Chap. 1), appears to be crucial for awareness and self-image, as well as to relate the perceptual and emotional selves to the external and internal environments (Devinsky 2009). The right hemisphere appears to contribute in important ways not only to the individual's relations to the external environment (through attention processes) but also to the processing of one's own identity and place in the world (Bartolomeo 2013).

Importantly, lesions in the opposite left hemisphere can also have consequences on bodily awareness but of a completely different sort. For example, when patients with left hemisphere damage are asked to point to the examiner's nose, they may instead indicate their own (heterotopoagnosia, Degos et al. 1997). Also, a typical consequence of left parietal (IPS) damage is the inability to recognize and name one's own fingers (finger agnosia), which with acalculia, agraphia, and left–right disorientation compose the so-called Gerstmann's syndrome (Rusconi et al. 2010).

Unfortunately, knowledge in the field of bodily related cognitive and emotional functions still lacks a systematic theoretical framework. Several models have been proposed, but none satisfactorily accounts for the available evidence from normal participants and brain-damaged patients (review in Berlucchi and Aglioti 2010). For example, Head and Holmes (1911) postulated the existence of two *body schemas*, one for the perception of posture or passive movement and another for the localization of stimuli on the skin. Analogous distinctions have been made between a *body schema*, seen as a nonconscious system of postural and sensorimotor capacities that usually functions without perceptual monitoring, and a *body image*, broadly envisaged as a set of perceptions, attitudes, and beliefs pertaining to one's own body as seen from the outside (Paillard 1999) and including the sense of ownership (Gallagher 2005). Another related proposal is a dichotomy between two somatosensory systems, one projecting to the PPC, dedicated to the immediate control of action, and another reaching the insula (Fig. 3.1), important for conscious perception and memory (Dijkerman and de Haan 2007). However, none of these frameworks seems sufficient to account for the dramatic hemispheric differences which are so evident in the clinical consequences of unilateral brain damage.

Visual perception of bodies induces specific changes in BOLD signals in normal participants in the middle fusiform gyrus (so-called fusiform body area or FBA) and in the right lateral occipitotemporal cortex (extrastriate body area, EBA, Fig. 3.1) (review in Peelen and Downing 2007). These regions are adjacent, but not identical, to the analogous occipitotemporal and mid-fusiform regions implicated in the visual perception of faces (Peelen and Downing 2007).

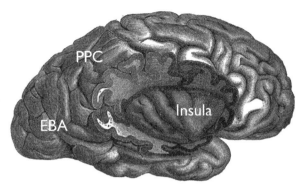

Fig. 3.1 Regions of the human right hemisphere important for body perception and awareness: the extrastriate body area (*EBA*), the posterior parietal cortex (*PPC*), and the anterior insula visible after removal of the opercula (Modified from Berlucchi and Aglioti (2010). © 2010, with permission from Springer)

3.2 Anosognosia and Anosodiaphoria

In 1914, Joseph Babinski coined the term *anosognosia* to describe the inability of being cognizant of hemiplegia in right-brain-damaged patients who were not otherwise confused (Babinski 1914). One of the patients reported in the original study had apparently normal intellectual and affective functions, but never complained about her left hemiplegia. When asked to move her right arm, she did so promptly; however, upon request to move her left arm, "she remained motionless and silent, behaving as if the question had been asked to another person" (Babinski 1914, p. 845). This condition did not depend on sensory problems, because the patient had impaired but present sensitivity to touch and passive motion of the left limbs. A second patient complained of a series of minor ailments, without ever mentioning her plegic left arm. When asked to move it, she did nothing and subsequently said, "here you are, it is done!" On the basis of the two cases he had described (but perhaps also of other cases he had observed in his clinical practice), Babinski wondered whether unawareness of the disease was specific to the lesions of the right hemisphere. Babinski also noted that other patients, without ignoring the existence of their paralysis, did not attach any importance to it, as if it were an insignificant disorder. He proposed to call *anosodiaphoria* this state of unconcern for the dramatic condition of being hemiplegic. For example, a patient with left hemiplegia reported by Critchley "replied in an almost facetious manner to requests that he should try and move the limbs … 'I can almost do it, but it just won't come.' He showed no distress and expressed no anxiety or even interest as to the chances of a return of power. Throughout the consultation, he cheerily and light-heartedly bandied small talk with his doctors" (Critchley 1953, p. 230f).

Josef Gerstmann provided a good description of a typical anosognosic patient: "The patient behaves as though he knew nothing about his hemiplegia, as though it had not existed, as though his paralyzed limbs were normal, and he insists that he can move them and can walk as well as he did before. Asked to lift up both arms, he naturally moves the healthy one only, but maintains that he has raised the disabled one also. Requests for movements with the paralyzed left arm or leg are performed by him merely with the healthy one, or not at all, but at the same time he is convinced that he has carried out the task. The patient may pay no attention to the paralyzed side, as though he had forgotten it; some not only neglect the defective side, but even refuse to look at it or turn away to the right. If such a patient is shown the affected arm or leg as being attached to his body, he will often remain indifferent or will declare that it is not his or that some one else's limb is in his bed, and the like. It is as though the patient experienced the paralyzed limbs as absent. Various illusions, distortions, confabulations and hallucinatory or delusional ideas may be produced in this connection" (Gerstmann 1942, p. 891f).

Although the original description of anosognosia concerned motor impairment, the term is now used to indicate unawareness of a variety of neurological deficits. These include somatosensory deficits such as hemianesthesia (again typically concerning the left side of the body of right-brain-damaged patients), visual field defects such as homonymous hemianopia or cerebral blindness (Anton's syndrome), memory deficits (e.g. in patients with Alzheimer's disease), and fluent aphasias (e.g., Wernicke's aphasia) resulting from post-Rolandic lesions of the left hemisphere.

Motor unawareness in brain-damaged patients remains, however, a major clinical problem, relatively common in the acute and postacute phase after a right hemisphere stroke. Its frequency varies in different studies; a meta-analysis estimated a frequency of anosognosia for hemiplegia in 54 % of patients after right hemisphere lesion and in 9 % after left hemisphere damage (Pia et al. 2004). Anosognosia for hemiplegia is understandably associated with a poorer outcome of rehabilitation and longer hospital stay, with the associated higher costs for patient management (Jenkinson et al. 2011). In one study (Gialanella and Mattioli 1992), anosognosia for hemiplegia turned out to be the worst prognostic factor for the motor and functional recovery from left hemiplegia due to stroke. In another study of 55 patients with right hemisphere stroke (Vossel et al. 2013), anosognosia for visuospatial deficits was the best predictor of impaired performance in standardized activities of daily living.

A simple, semiquantitative score of anosognosia (Bisiach et al. 1986) takes the following values: 0 (spontaneous complaint by the patient), 1 (the patient acknowledges his/her impairment following a specific question by the examiner), 2 (the disorder is acknowledged upon demonstration through standard neurological examination), and 3 (no acknowledgment is possible). Other scales (e.g., Azouvi et al. 2003, see Sect. 4.8) compare scores obtained from the patient to scores provided by the caregiver. These scores typically dissociate in the case of anosognosia, because the patient tends to provide more optimistic results than the caregiver.

In a study of 58 patients with right hemisphere damage (Vocat et al. 2010), anosognosia of hemiplegia was frequent (32 %) in the hyperacute phase 3 days after the stroke, but substantially decreased 1 week later (18 %) and became rare at 6 months (5 %). There were double dissociations between anosognosia and proprioceptive impairments or visual neglect (see Chap. 4). The first dissociation militates against Babinski's early hypothesis of sensory deafferentation as a major determinant of anosognosia (Babinski 1914). However, scores for

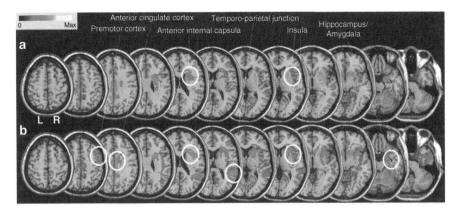

Fig. 3.2 Voxel-based lesion mapping of anosognosia for left hemiplegia. Brain regions where damage was significantly related to the severity of anosognosia for hemiplegia in the hyperacute phase (**a**) and in the subacute phase (**b**). The voxels *highlighted* are those that show a significant difference (*t* > 2.7, *P* < 0.01, false discovery rate corrected) in the composite scores of anosognosia for hemiplegia between patients with or without a lesion in these voxels. *L* left, *R* right (Reproduced from Vocat et al. (2010). © 2010, with permission from Oxford University Press)

proprioceptive deficits and neglect strongly correlated with scores of anosognosia, raising the possibility that impaired proprioception might well be a contributing factor to this condition, for example, by impairing the patient's "appreciation" of the current state of the paralyzed limb (Levine 1990; Vuilleumier 2004). Vocat et al. (2010) performed a voxel-based statistical mapping (see Sect. 7.2), which highlighted damage to the insula (see also Karnath et al. 2005) and adjacent sub-cortical structures in the hyperacute period. Additional lesions were associated with the persistence of anosognosia for hemiplegia in the subacute phase after 1 week from stroke. These regions were likely to suffer from ischemic penumbra without structural damage in patients who recovered from anosognosia after a few days. These additional lesions were located in the premotor cortex (see also Berti et al. 2005), the dorsal ACC, the TPJ, and the medial temporal structures (hippocampus and amygdala) (Fig. 3.2). Vocat et al. (2010) concluded that anosognosia is likely to depend on damage to a distributed set of brain regions, resulting in multiple coexisting deficits, such as impaired sensation, attention, interoceptive bodily representations, motor programming, error monitoring, and memory and affective processing, possibly with different combinations in different patients.

3.3 Misoplegia and Left Hemiconcern

Much more rarely, patients with right hemisphere damage may show signs of morbid dislike, aversion, and even hostility towards the affected left side of the body, a disturbance dubbed "misoplegia" by Macdonald Critchley (1974).

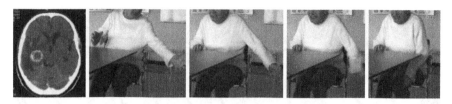

Fig. 3.3 Misoplegia without hemiplegia. In a patient with a gliosarcoma affecting the right temporal and parietal lobes. Here is a transcript of the dialogue between the examiner and the patient. Examiner: What's the matter with your leg, I noticed you're beating your leg? Patient: Yes, this happens every now and then. (The patient starts beating her left leg) You bugger, you damn bugger! You are not even able to pick up that slipper. E: That means you also call it by name? P: Yes, I call it "bugger" (Reproduced from Loetscher et al. (2006). © 2006, with permission from BMJ Publishing Group Ltd.)

In the works of Critchley, "occasionally we find a patient displaying a veritable dislike of the paralysed limbs which evoke feelings of disgust, dismay, and even horror. The paralysed arm may be kept covered by the bedclothes or a shawl so as to conceal it. Or the patient may keep the gaze averted from the affected side..." (Critchley 1955, p. 286). Patients can personify their plegic limbs and call them names or even hit them with the good hand. A motor deficit is not invariably present. Critchley (1979) described the case of a patient with mild hemiparesis but severe loss of postural sensitivity and hemianopia, who addressed his left arm as follows: "You bloody bastard! ... It keeps following me around. It gets in my way when I read. I find my hand up by my face, waving about." Loetscher et al. (2006) reported on a patient with a grade IV gliosarcoma in a patient with a gliosarcoma affecting the right temporal and parietal lobes (Fig. 3.3). She had no motor deficit, but used to strike her left leg violently, calling it names.

Critchley (1979) reports on patients who have called their paralyzed arms "George," "Toby," "silly Billy," "the immovable one," "the curse," "lazy boy," "old useless," "floppy Joe," "little monkey," "the delinquent," and "the communist" (in relation to the arm's refusal to work). Other patients may develop illusions concerning the size and appearance of the affected limb, which may be assimilated to a bird's claw, a "heavy iron bar," "a piece of dead meat," and "the hand of a mummy" (Critchley 1979).

In contrast to this disturbance, Bogousslavsky et al. (1995) coined the term *acute hemiconcern* to describe three patients in the acute phase of a stroke in the territory of the right anterior parietal artery (postcentral gyrus, parts or superior and middle temporal gyri, anterior part of inferior parietal gyrus, and supramarginal gyrus) with severe somatosensory and proprioceptive loss. These patients showed an exceedingly caring attitude towards their left limbs, looking at them for long periods, and relentlessly manipulating parts of their left hemisoma with their right hand or foot. This behavior receded within a few days. The authors proposed that hyperexploration of the left hemisoma would result from a feeling of estrangement from the body parts affected by the sensory loss in the absence of neglect. However, none of 13 patients with mirror-image lesions in the left hemisphere demonstrated such behavior, suggesting that the feeling of estrangement must somehow depend on right hemisphere damage.

3.4 Asomatognosia and Somatoparaphrenia

Patients with right hemisphere damage may develop peculiar and dramatic disturbances of awareness of the left half of their body. *Asomatognosia* was defined by
Critchley (1953) as the "loss of awareness of one body-half." Patients may deny or
be confused about the presence and ownership of their left limbs, for example, by
mistaking their left arm for the examiner's. The problem may in some cases be corrected either by verbally convincing the patient of the ownership of his/her limbs or
by the patients' use of their right hand to follow the left arm up to the shoulder.

Some patients produce confabulatory accounts of their left limbs. For example,
one of the patients reported by Feinberg et al. (2010) repeatedly talked of "a hand
that was left on the subway and they brought it here and they put it on me"; another
said, "It's supposed to be my arm, but I think it's my brother's arm. I tell that to
everyone but they don't believe me. My brother was on the wrong track for a while,
and he got involved with some gangsters. They chopped off his arms and threw
them in the river. I found this in my coffin. (Touching the left arm) Some people
thought I was dead, and it was there. I don't know why I was in a coffin... after I
was carried to the hospital... I was in a coffin... that's what I remember... I was
laying next to this arm (pointing to left arm)... I was in a coffin... Yeah that's how
I found it. I was alive... I didn't die... I found the arm in the coffin."

When asomatognosia is accompanied by these elaborate and articulate delusional aspects and is refractory to the examiner's demonstrations, the term *somatoparaphrenia* (Gerstmann 1942) is often employed. These patients firmly believe
that their left limbs do not belong to them (feelings of disownership) or that they
belong to someone else. A patient suffering from such a delusion was described by
Jean-Baptiste Bouillaud (1825), long before the condition was recognized as a typical consequence of right hemisphere lesions: "The left side [of his body] was so
insensitive, that the patient regarded it as if it were a stranger to him; it seemed to
him that somebody else's body was lying on his side, or even a corpse. This peculiar
sensitive illusion was the principal object of his daydreaming since his stroke.
Requested to move his left limbs, he moved his right limbs instead" (p. 64). Another
patient described by Hermann Zingerle (1913) "continued to report that to the left
of himself a woman was lying in the bed, and, in the meantime, he pointed to the
left, and it was impossible to make him refrain from this, even by visual exploration
[of the left side of space]. He often reported this impression combined with erotic
joking, caressing his left arm. Yet, at the same time, he also complained about the
inconvenience which it caused to him, particularly during the night hours; he was
insensitive to passive movements. At this time, conversation with him on this topic
took a very strange course. Whereas nothing unusual was noticed when talking to
the patient about everyday matters or about his other physical conditions, and
whereas he followed promptly and correctly commands regarding his right arm and
leg, or to show his tongue, he suddenly failed and appeared grossly perplexed when
one started to talk about the left side of his body, or asked questions concerning it.
He appeared embarrassed, looked for an excuse, became mute and inattentive, and

it was also impossible to evoke old memories of his left side. The same happened when the physician demonstrated the left side on his [the patient's] own body. He knew it: but this knowledge was irrelevant for his own person, and could clarify nothing. If one insisted, trying to make clear the discrepancies between his strange perceptions and reality by way of instruction, or guidance of his gaze, he became progressively agitated and absolutely unable to appreciate the situation. He was unaware of the oddity and absurdity of having only a right half" (English translation by Benke et al. 2004). The delusion receded after 2 weeks, when the patient started to acknowledge that his body had a left side and that it was paralyzed.

In a more recent multiple case report (Gandola et al. 2012), another right-brain-damaged patient stated: "No, it's not my hand… it is yours." "It occupies a lot of space in this bed, it's so uncomfortable." "It is an artificial limb… not mine… it is of the nurse… it is very intrusive, I've no more space in this bed!" "Yes, please take it away… I don't care about its destiny as it is not mine." In most cases the delusion is associated with motor anosognosia (but there are occasional cases without anosognosia) and visual neglect. It is typically transient, lasting a few days after the occurrence of right hemispheric strokes, often involving subcortical white matter, basal ganglia, and thalamus (Gandola et al. 2012). However, a patient under the care of Jean-Denis Degos (1997, personal communication) after dismissal from the hospital wrote to the hospital director to complain that, despite having been very well cared for, the personnel had had the bad taste of putting a cadaver in his bed!

It is important to note that these patients do not have generalized delirium or delusional beliefs, except those concerning the left side of their left body. *Misoplegia* (see the preceding section) may be considered to belong to this spectrum of disorders characterized by feelings of disownership of the left limbs, treated as foreign objects, sometimes with deprecatory remarks. These disorders of bodily awareness are typically accompanied by proprioceptive deficits and left visual neglect; anosognosia for hemiplegia is often, but not always, present (Vallar and Ronchi 2009).

Damage to a variety of right hemisphere sites has been associated with asomatognosia and somatoparaphrenia. Vallar and Ronchi (2009) cite several cases with extensive fronto–temporoparietal damage. In other cases, the lesion was more localized, often in the supramarginal gyrus of the IPL and underlying white matter. Still other patients had lesions in the insula, basal ganglia, thalamus, subcortical white matter, or in the territory of the anterior cerebral artery (cingulate gyrus, supplementary motor area, genu of the corpus callosum).

3.5 Supernumerary Phantom Limbs, Xenomelia, and Autoscopic Phenomena

In rare cases, patients with right hemisphere damage may develop disorders reminiscent of amputees' "phantom limbs." They may feel the presence of one or more supernumerary limbs, just as amputees or patients with brachial plexus lesions may feel the presence of the amputated or insensitive limb. A patient reported by

Halligan et al. (1993), who had developed left hemiplegia and sensory loss after the occurrence of a large cerebral hematoma in the right basal ganglia region, sometimes denied ownership of his left arm and leg, saying that they had been amputated 23 years before. On subsequent testing he showed no signs of anosognosia or anosodiaphoria, revealing normal insight and concern about the effects of his brain lesion. However, he firmly believed that he owned a third arm, which he claimed originated from the top left corner of his torso. This belief held for several months. Here follow some excerpts from his interviews. Examiner: "What can you not do at the moment?" Patient: "I can't use my left hand or my left side… I can't do anything with them … it's a terrible stroke condition… it's like a sack of coal … I'm like an unguided missile… I fall all over the place." However, when asked specifically if there was something special about his hand, he answered: "Yes, I have a third one." Examiner: "A third one?" Patient: "Yes." Examiner: "Where is that?" Patient: "It is in the middle" (…) Examiner: "So tell me now at the moment, how many hands do you have?" Patient: "Three" (…). Examiner: "Count the number of hands you have for me." Patient (looking down and pointing): "… One… two… three." The patient's description of his third limb as having the thumb on the right side with the palm facing down suggests that the phantom limb was a left arm. The patient did not feel comfortable with his phantom limb belief; on one occasion he commented, "I know it's a nonsense" and began to show signs of agitation, which brought the interview to an end.

Cipriani et al. (2011) described another patient, who repeatedly reported that he had a third arm protruding from his left elbow. He was astonished by this feeling and recognized that it did not correspond to reality. CT scan showed a small low-density area in the right TPJ. Also this patient had signs of left neglect and sensory loss in his left arm. Two months later, the phantom limb feeling had disappeared, but the patient retained the memory of the illusion and was still amazed by it.

Madame S, studied by Bourlon et al. (2012), was a 58-year-old woman with left hemiparesis, superficial and deep sensory deficits in the left upper limb, and signs of left visual neglect consequent to the occurrence of an intracerebral hematoma in the right hemisphere (Fig. 3.4a). Madame S reported phantom feelings of movement and warmth in her upper left limb, which gave her the impression of having a third hand (Fig. 3.4b). She could not "see" the phantom hand and was well aware of the illusory character of this impression. The illusion lasted for more than 1 year.

The term *xenomelia* (McGeoch et al. 2011) denotes another rare condition featuring an abnormal attitude towards one's limbs. Patients with xenomelia have the oppressive feeling that one or more limbs of one's body do not belong to one's self and insistently demand that the "foreign" limb be amputated. At variance with all the previously described conditions, xenomelia is not apparently related to acquired brain damage; there may be no neurological or psychiatric abnormalities. However, there are hints that a right hemisphere dysfunction participates in the occurrence of xenomelia (McGeoch et al. 2011). The estranged limb is frequently a lower left limb, and recent MRI evidence demonstrated reduced cortical thickness in the SPL and reduced cortical surface area in the primary and secondary somatosensory cortices, in the IPL, and in the anterior insular cortex in the right hemisphere (Hilti et al. 2013).

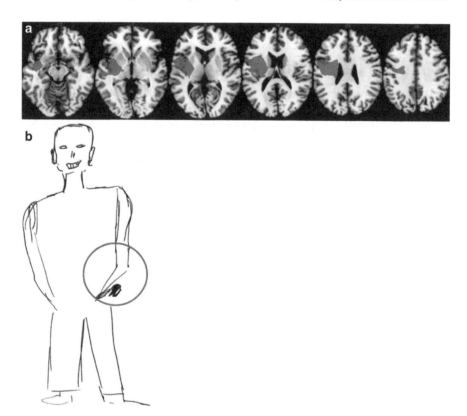

Fig. 3.4 (**a**) Schematic reconstruction of Madame S's lesion, implicating the frontal lobe (pre- and postcentral gyrus, Rolandic operculum, inferior frontal gyrus), the superior temporal gyrus and the Heschl gyri, the insula, and the basal ganglia (caudate, putamen, pallidum). The right hemisphere is on the *left side* of the scans. (**b**) Madame S's rendering of the position of her third hand (*circled in red*)

Patients with *autoscopic hallucinations* see an image of their own body as if they were looking into a mirror, but without identifying themselves with the hallucinated body. Patients often hallucinate their own face or the upper part of the trunk. There are often other visual hallucinations or visual illusions and visual field deficits. Autoscopic hallucinations have been associated with lesions of the right occipital or occipitoparietal cortex. Heydrich and Blanke (2013) described a right hemisphere lesion in six out of seven patients with autoscopic hallucinations. Lesions overlapped on the right occipital cortex, more specifically the superior occipital gyrus and the cuneus in extrastriate visual cortex. The damaged territory likely included the EBA, the FBA, and the fusiform face area (see above Sect. 3.2).

Distinct forms of autoscopic phenomena include *out-of-body experiences*, whereby one's own body is seen from an elevated perspective, and *heautoscopy*, characterized by strong self-identification with one's own second body, often associated with a duplication of the subject's experience of the world, as if he or she were existing in two places at the same time. The right TPJ seems to be implicated in bodily self-consciousness and out-of-body experiences (Ionta et al. 2011). Heydrich and Blanke (2013) reported damage to the left temporal lobe and/or left insula in seven patients with heautoscopy.

3.6 Motor Impersistence

Fisher (1956) defined *motor impersistence* as the inability to maintain in time a given posture, such as closing the eyes, protruding the tongue, or keeping the mouth open, and linked its occurrence to right hemisphere lesions. Kertesz et al. (1985) confirmed the increased frequency of motor impersistence after right hemisphere damage, especially in the frontal lobe. The most discriminating tests were eye closure, mouth opening, tongue protrusion, and gaze to the left. They related this phenomenon to mechanisms of directed attention that are necessary to sustain motor activity.

Failure to keep the eyes closed was the most common manifestation of motor impersistence in the series described by De Renzi et al. (1986). Sakai et al. (2000) explored 160 stroke patients and found simultanapraxia (the inability to perform two motor acts simultaneously: closing the eyes and protruding the tongue) associated to motor impersistence in nine patients (5.6 %). Typical MRI lesions included areas 6 and 8 and the underlying subcortical white matter in the territory of the right middle cerebral artery. Seo et al. (2007) described a case of right medial frontal lobe lesions with callosal disconnection (genu and body). After the stroke, the patient showed left limb hypokinesia and right limb motor impersistence. Thus, inadequate transmission of information between the right hemisphere and the left motor areas may result in motor impersistence.

References

Azouvi P, Olivier S, de Montety G, Samuel C, Louis-Dreyfus A, Tesio L. Behavioral assessment of unilateral neglect: study of the psychometric properties of the Catherine Bergego Scale. Arch Phys Med Rehabil. 2003;84:51–7.

Babinski J. Contribution à l'étude des troubles mentaux dans l'hémiplégie organique (anosognosie). Revue Neurol. 1914;27:845–8.

Bartolomeo P. The Delusion of the Master: the last days of Henry James. Neurological Sciences. 2013;34:2031–4.

Benke T, Luzzatti C, Vallar G. Hermann Zingerle's "Impaired perception of the own body due to organic brain disorders". 1913. An introductory comment, and an abridged translation. Cortex. 2004;40:265–74.

Berlucchi G, Aglioti SM. The body in the brain revisited. Exp Brain Res. 2010;200:25–35.

Berti A, Bottini G, Gandola M, Pia L, Smania N, Stracciari A, Castiglioni I, Vallar G, Paulesu E. Shared cortical anatomy for motor awareness and motor control. Science. 2005;309:488–91.

Bisiach E, Vallar G, Perani D, Papagno C, Berti A. Unawareness of disease following lesions of the right hemisphere: anosognosia for hemiplegia and anosognosia for hemianopia. Neuropsychologia. 1986;24:471–82.

Bogousslavsky J, Kumral E, Regli F, Assal G, Ghika J. Acute hemiconcern: a right anterior parietotemporal syndrome. J Neurol Neurosurg Psychiatry. 1995;58:428–32.

Bouillaud J.-B. Traité clinique et physiologique de l'encéphalite, ou inflammation du cerveau, et de ses suites. Paris: Chez J.-B. Baillière; 1825.

Bourlon C, Bourgeois A, Vandier J, Bordier A, Baradji M, Bartolomeo P, Duret C. Membre fantôme surnuméraire: le cas de Madame S. Rev Neurol. 2012;168:A21–2.

Cipriani G, Picchi L, Vedovello M, Nuti A, Fiorino MD. The phantom and the supernumerary phantom limb: historical review and new case. Neurosci Bull. 2011;27:359–65.

Critchley M. The parietal lobes. New York: Hafner; 1953.

Critchley M. Personification of paralysed limbs in hemiplegics. Br Med J. 1955;2:284–6.

Critchley M. Misoplegia, or hatred of hemiplegia. Mount Sinai J Med. 1974;41:82–7.

Critchley M. Misoplegia, or hatred of hemiplegia. In: The divine banquet of the brain. New York: Raven Press; 1979. p. 115–20.

De Renzi E, Gentilini M, Bazolli C. Eyelid movement disorders and motor impersistence in acute hemisphere disease. Neurology. 1986;36:414–18.

Degos JD, Bachoud-Levi AC, Ergis AM, Petrissans JL, Cesaro P. Selective inability to point to extrapersonal targets after left posterior parietal lesions: an objectivization disorder? Neurocase. 1997;3:31–9.

Devinsky O. Delusional misidentifications and duplications: right brain lesions, left brain delusions. Neurology. 2009;72:80–7.

Dijkerman HC, de Haan EH. Somatosensory processes subserving perception and action. Behav Brain Sci. 2007;30:189–201; discussion 201–39.

Feinberg T, Keenan J. Where in the brain is the self? Conscious Cogn. 2005;14:661–78.

Feinberg TE, Venneri A, Simone AM, Fan Y, Northoff G. The neuroanatomy of asomatognosia and somatoparaphrenia. J Neurol Neurosurg Psychiatry. 2010;81:276–81.

Fisher M. Left hemiplegia and motor impersistence. J Nerv Ment Dis. 1956;123:201–18.

Gallagher S. How the body shapes the mind. New York: Oxford University Press; 2005.

Gandola M, Invernizzi P, Sedda A, Ferre ER, Sterzi R, Sberna M, Paulesu E, Bottini G. An anatomical account of somatoparaphrenia. Cortex. 2012;48:1165–78.

Gerstmann J. Problem of imperception of disease and of impaired body territories with organic lesions: relation to body scheme and its disorders. Arch Neurol Psychiatry. 1942;48:890–913.

Gialanella B, Mattioli F. Anosognosia and extrapersonal neglect as predictors of functional recovery following right hemisphere stroke. Neuropsychol Rehabil. 1992;2:169–78.

Halligan PW, Marshall JC, Wade DT. Three arms: a case study of supernumerary phantom limb after right hemisphere stroke. J Neurol Neurosurg Psychiatry. 1993;56:159–66.

Head H, Holmes G. Sensory disturbances from cerebral lesion. Brain. 1911;34:102–254.

Hervé P-Y, Zago L, Petit L, Mazoyer B, Tzourio-Mazoyer N. Revisiting human hemispheric specialization with neuroimaging. Trends Cogn Sci. 2013;17(2):69–80.

Heydrich L, Blanke O. Distinct illusory own-body perceptions caused by damage to posterior insula and extrastriate cortex. Brain. 2013;136:790–803.

Hilti LM, Jr H, Vitacco DA, Kraemer B, Palla A, Luechinger R, Jäncke L, Brugger P. The desire for healthy limb amputation: structural brain correlates and clinical features of xenomelia. Brain. 2013;136:318–29.

Ionta S, Heydrich L, Lenggenhager B, Mouthon M, Fornari E, Chapuis D, Gassert R, Blanke O. Multisensory mechanisms in temporo-parietal cortex support self-location and first-person perspective. Neuron. 2011;70:363–74.

James W. The principles of psychology. New York: Henry Holt; 1890.

Jenkinson PM, Preston C, Ellis SJ. Unawareness after stroke: a review and practical guide to understanding, assessing, and managing anosognosia for hemiplegia. J Clin Exp Neuropsychol. 2011;33:1079–93.

Karnath HO, Baier B, Nagele T. Awareness of the functioning of one's own limbs mediated by the insular cortex? J Neurosci. 2005;25:7134–8.

Kertesz A, Nicholson I, Cancelliere A, Kassa K, Black SE. Motor impersistence: a right-hemisphere syndrome. Neurology. 1985;35:662–6.

Lee K, Shinbo M, Kanai H, Nagumo Y. Reduplicative paramnesia after a right frontal lesion. Cogn Behav Neurol. 2011;24:35–9.

Levine DN. Unawareness of visual and sensorimotor defects: a hypothesis. Brain Cogn. 1990;13:233–81.

Loetscher T, Regard M, Brugger P. Misoplegia: a review of the literature and a case without hemiplegia. J Neurol Neurosurg Psychiatry. 2006;77:1099–100.

McGeoch PD, Brang D, Song T, Lee RR, Huang M, Ramachandran VS. Xenomelia: a new right parietal lobe syndrome. J Neurol Neurosurg Psychiatry. 2011;82:1314–19.

Paillard J. Body schema and body image—a double dissociation in deafferented patients. In: Gantchev GN, Mori S, Massion J, editors. Motor control, today and tomorrow. Sofia: Academic Publishing House; 1999.

Peelen MV, Downing PE. The neural basis of visual body perception. Nat Rev Neurosci. 2007;8:636–48.

Pia L, Neppi-Modona M, Ricci R, Berti A. The anatomy of anosognosia for hemiplegia: a meta-analysis. Cortex. 2004;40:367–77.

Rusconi E, Pinel P, Dehaene S, Kleinschmidt A. The enigma of Gerstmann's syndrome revisited: a telling tale of the vicissitudes of neuropsychology. Brain. 2010;133:320–32.

Sakai Y, Nakamura T, Sakurai A, Yamaguchi H, Hirai S. Right frontal areas 6 and 8 are associated with simultanapraxia, a subset of motor impersistence. Neurology. 2000;54:522–4.

Seo SW, Jung K, You H, Kim EJ, Lee BH, Adair JC, Na DL. Dominant limb motor impersistence associated with callosal disconnection. Neurology. 2007;68:862–4.

Vallar G, Ronchi R. Somatoparaphrenia: a body delusion. A review of the neuropsychological literature. Exp Brain Res. 2009;192:533–51.

Vocat R, Staub F, Stroppini T, Vuilleumier P. Anosognosia for hemiplegia: a clinical-anatomical prospective study. Brain. 2010;133:3578–97.

Vossel S, Weiss PH, Eschenbeck P, Fink GR. Anosognosia, neglect, extinction and lesion site predict impairment of daily living after right-hemispheric stroke. Cortex. 2013;49:1782–9.

Vuilleumier P. Anosognosia: the neurology of beliefs and uncertainties. Cortex. 2004;40:9–17.

Zingerle H. Über Störungen der Wahrnehmung des eigenen Körpers bei organischen Gehirnerkrankungen. Monatsschr Psychiatr Neurol. 1913;34:13–36.

Further Reading

Berlucchi G, Aglioti SM. The body in the brain revisited. Exp Brain Res. 2010;200(1):25–35.

Critchley M. The parietal lobes. New York: Hafner; 1953.

Vallar G, Ronchi R. Somatoparaphrenia: a body delusion. A review of the neuropsychological literature. Exp Brain Res. 2009;192(3):533–51.

Chapter 4
Unilateral Spatial Neglect: Clinical Aspects

Keywords Spatial cognition • Reading • Target search • Line bisection • Drawing tasks • Representational tasks

4.1 Definition and Causes

Unilateral spatial neglect has been defined as the inability to detect, respond to, and orient towards novel and significant stimuli occurring in the half space contralateral to a brain lesion (Heilman and Valenstein 1979). This definition was subsequently accepted by most authors, with the addition of a definitional criterion and of an important observation (Gainotti et al. 2008). The criterion excludes from the definition of neglect the visuospatial disorders that can be considered as a simple consequence of elementary sensorimotor disorders (such as visual field defects, see Sect. 2.1), which are often present in patients with brain damage. The observation is that neglect signs are much more frequent and more severe after right hemispheric lesions and, therefore, in typical cases neglect affects the left half of space (Gainotti 1968; Vallar and Perani 1986; Halligan et al. 1989). Right neglect after left hemisphere damage is much less common, severe, and durable (Beis et al. 2004). Moreover, some damage to right hemisphere attention systems (perhaps particularly to those implicated in alertness, see Sect. 1.2) might be necessary for signs of right neglect to emerge in left-brain-damaged patients (Weintraub et al. 1996; Bartolomeo et al. 1998; Andrade et al. 2010).

However, as noted by Gainotti et al. (2008), the classical definition of neglect does not completely account for the complexity of its manifestations. First, this definition suggests that peripersonal space is divided into two halves by a plane corresponding to the patient's midsagittal plane and that one of these halves is neglected by the patient. In fact, the distinction between the right half and the left half of space must be seen in a relative and dynamic way rather than a static and absolute one. Indeed, neglect patients do not necessarily neglect all of the objects on the left side of their body midsagittal plane (Marshall and Halligan 1989a), they may in fact neglect a stimulus situated to the relative left of another (left- or right-sided) stimulus or ignore the left side of several stimuli, regardless of their absolute location in the visual scene (see Sect. 6.1.4). Thus, the prefix "hemi-" in widely used terms such as "hemispatial neglect," "hemineglect," or "hemi-inattention" does not seem entirely representative of the full range of phenomena encountered.

Second, this definition implies that neglect is a single, homogeneous nosologic entity, whose manifestations essentially result from the spatial location of stimuli and much less so from the nature of the task. In fact, on the one hand, the nature of the task appears to play a significant role in the development of the manifestations of neglect; for example, well-identified variables (such as the amount of general attentional load or the presence of distracting stimuli on the "good" side) can predict whether the left half of a given item will be neglected or not by the patient (see, e.g., Bartolomeo et al. 2004). On the other hand, neglect does not seem to be a homogeneous disorder, but may appear selectively as a function of several variables including (1) the nature and difficulty of the requested activities (e.g., perceptual, motor, or representational); (2) the spatial sector involved in the task (personal (located on the body), peripersonal (near), or extrapersonal (far)), which might well rely on partly distinct brain systems (Rizzolatti et al. 1983; Colby and Goldberg 1999); and (3) the nature of the spatial coordinates (ego- or object-centered) used for apprehending the relevant material.

Third, the current definition only considers the negative aspect of the syndrome (i.e., neglect for stimuli located on the left), with no notice of the positive aspects, which could be at the forefront in the most severe manifestations of neglect, such as the tendency to automatically (or "magnetically") orient attention to stimuli on the right side of space or the tendency that some patients show to perseverate in checking stimuli presented on the "good," non-neglected side. Finally, although lateralized spatial deficits are immediately apparent from the clinical point of view, the important role of non-lateralized aspects of neglect has been repeatedly stressed (Robertson 2001). As a consequence, even the attribute "unilateral" has been criticized concerning neglect.

The cause of neglect is most often vascular strokes, but signs of neglect may also be observed as a consequence of brain tumors (Hughlings Jackson 1876/1932) or of neurodegenerative conditions, such as Alzheimer's disease (Bartolomeo et al. 1998) and posterior cortical atrophy (Andrade et al. 2010, 2012). Given the growing prevalence of neurodegenerative conditions with increasing life expectancy in Western countries, these causes of neglect are likely to progressively become more of a clinical concern (see Chap. 8).

4.2 Clinical Presentation

In a similar way to aphasic deficits after left brain damage, neglect is a frequent set of disabling signs and symptoms that have dramatic implications in the daily lives of patients.

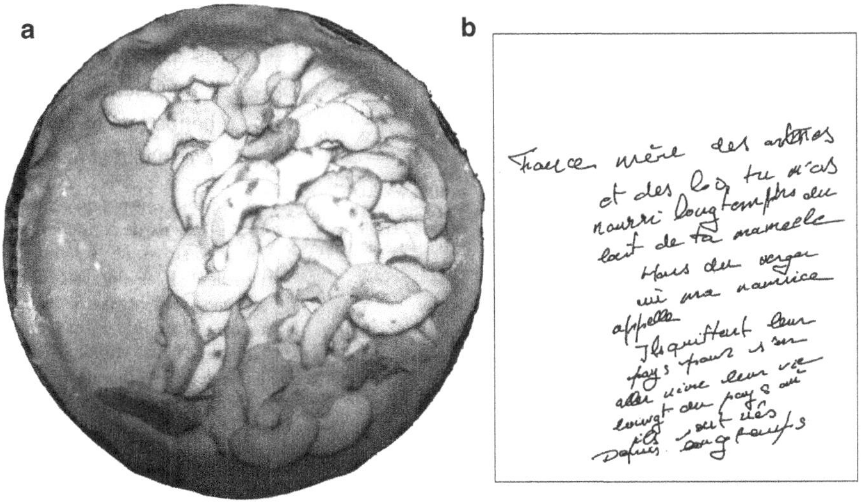

Fig. 4.1 (**a**) An apple pie made by a patient with left neglect. (**b**) Spontaneous writing (Reproduced from Rode et al. (2007), Fig. 10.1. © 2007, with permission from Oxford University Press)

In the most severe forms, especially in the acute phase of vascular lesions affecting the territory of the right middle cerebral artery, the presence of neglect can be inferred only from patients' spontaneous behavior, since any formal investigation is practically impossible. In this case, it is essentially the posture of patients which is clinically suggestive. They remain in their beds, keeping the head and eyes deviated to the side opposite to their hemiplegia (see Sect. 2.4), and do not respond to stimuli from the neglected side of space.

Any incentive to engage in a task with a spatial component exaggerates the gaze deviation, which tends to cling to objects at the far right of the visual field. In the days following the acute phase, the lateral deviation of the eyes diminishes and disappears gradually, but a tendency to "magnetically" look at stimuli located to the right of the patient remains clear and can typically be highlighted when the visual field of patients are assessed with the method of confrontation described above (see Sect. 2.2).

With the gradual disappearance of the postural bias, it becomes possible to observe typical behavioral manifestations, both during activities that the patient performs with his/her body and in response to stimuli from the external environment. Typical manifestations of personal or bodily neglect (Sect. 4.7.2) are the tendency to wash, shave, comb, or dress only the right half of the body. Patients may forget to wear the left sleeve or slipper and leave hanging the left earpiece of their spectacles (Nicklason and Finucane 1990). Behavioral signs of extrapersonal neglect are the tendency to eat only the food in the right half of the plate and read only the right half of the journal titles, despite the consequent lack of sense (*neglect dyslexia*, see Sect. 4.4.4 below). At this stage, when questioned from the left side, patients may refrain from responding, or they may answer another person standing on their right side. Thus, neglect signs can be apparent in everyday activities, such as cooking or writing (Fig. 4.1).

When patients can perform neuropsychological tests (Sect. 4.3), they show signs of severe left unilateral neglect, with performance often confined to a restricted region of the right hemispace, without reaching the sagittal midline. Patients who are able to stand often demonstrate disorders of postural control, perhaps related to neglect of graviceptive, somesthetic, vestibular, and visual information (Perennou 2006).

The clinical picture of neglect often develops in a set of signs and symptoms typically observed in extensive lesions of the right sylvian region, in the territory of the middle cerebral artery. More rarely, left neglect develops after more ventral lesions, such as strokes in the territory of the posterior cerebral artery (see Chap. 7). Another rare occurrence is right-sided neglect after left hemisphere damage, which is usually less severe than left neglect and recovers more rapidly, except in the case of progressive disorders such as neurodegenerative diseases (Bartolomeo et al. 1998).

The following signs can be observed: (1) disturbances of relatively elementary sensorimotor functions such as hemiplegia or hemiparesis, left oculomotor disorders, left homonymous hemianopia, and extinction of left events on double simultaneous stimulation in one or more sensory modalities (see Chap. 2); (2) unilateral disturbances of bodily cognition, such as asomatognosia, motor neglect, somatoparaphrenia, and anosognosia (see Chap. 3); (3) disorders of emotional behavior, ranging from anosodiaphoria to the tendency to make puns (or sometimes misoplegia; see Chap. 3) and to disturbances in emotional recognition and expression (somatic or vegetative); (4) signs of impaired diffuse attention functions, with general slowing of behavior and motor manifestations of motor impersistence (Sect. 3.6); (5) so-called "apraxic" disorders (constructional apraxia and dressing apraxia); and (6) variable non-lateralized spatial deficits, such as impaired spatial analysis and visuospatial exploration characterized by erratic search strategies (Weintraub and Mesulam 1988).

Following the first few days after the stroke, patients may recover from gross behavioral signs of neglect in everyday life. In this phase, diagnosis of neglect rests on appropriate neuropsychological testing, in which patients may be able to attend to information from the right half of the display sheet but still show defective performance on the left side.

After a period ranging from weeks to months since lesion onset, a substantial proportion of patients may learn to compensate for neglect both in everyday life and in paper-and-pencil tasks. Even in these "recovered" patients, however, subtler signs of spatial bias can be demonstrated. Patients continue to begin their exploration from the right side (Mattingley et al. 1994b), whereas most normal individuals use a left-to-right scanning technique, possibly due to reading habits (Chokron and Imbert 1993). When producing a manual or vocal response to lateralized visual targets, patients respond more slowly to left than to right targets, especially at the beginning of the test (Bartolomeo 1997), as if a residual initial attraction for right-sided objects were at work (Mattingley et al. 1994b). Thus, the use of appropriate, often computer-based tasks with emphasis on RTs, can unmask residual signs of spatial bias in patients who have apparently recovered from signs of neglect on paper-and-pencil tests (Bonato 2012). This has clinical implications, because these patients should not be allowed to engage in activities requiring fast reactions to external stimuli, such as for example driving (see Sect. 4.3).

However, a number of patients do not recover from behavioral signs of neglect. For these patients, the presence of neglect may affect negatively motor recovery (Denes et al. 1982). Thus, neglect does not only have important implications for understanding the brain mechanisms of space processing, it also constitutes a major clinical problem.

4.3   Diagnostic Tests: General Considerations

When the behavioral manifestations of neglect, with complete neglect for everything that is not located at the extreme right of the patient, have faded and patients are again able to freely distribute their attention on less limited spatial areas, it becomes possible to use standardized methods of examination to make a more formal assessment of neglect signs. A few paper-and-pencil tests, easily administrable at the patient's bedside, can assess the presence and severity of several neglect signs. Standardized batteries including several sorts of these tests are currently available (Halligan et al. 1989; Azouvi et al. 2006). Schematically, neuropsychological tasks for neglect assessment can be distinguished in visuo-perceptual tests, visuo-graphic tests, and representational (or imaginal) tests (Gainotti et al. 2008). Signs of neglect can occur in nonvisual sensory modalities such as the auditory and tactile modalities, but they are generally milder and not often assessed in clinical practice (Bartolomeo and Chokron 2001; Gainotti 2010).

As a general point when administering paper-and-pencil tasks in spatially-based disorders such as neglect, care should be taken in the proper positioning of the test sheet. In the usual clinical conditions, the vertical midline of the sheet should be approximately aligned with the midsagittal plane of the trunk of the patient. The patient should not be allowed to displace the sheet during the test; to this end, the sheet can be attached to the desk by using transparent adhesive tape, or the examiner can hold a central part of the sheet (Fig. 4.2). A second general point is that the examiner should avoid giving spatial cues to the patient during testing, such as, for example, pointing at a target during visual search tasks.

Importantly, as mentioned in the preceding section, patients who perform normally on paper-and-pencil tests may nevertheless show spatial or nonspatial deficits on more stringent tests of visuospatial attention, such as speeded RT tests. It is important to be aware of the possibility of these "subclinical" deficits, which might well have clinical implications, for example, in taking decisions about the patient's ability to drive. Cases in which patients are able to compensate for their deficits on paper-and-pencil tests, but nevertheless show RT asymmetries, visual extinction, or other subtle signs of spatial bias, might put the patient and other people at risk in situations requiring rapid reactions to external stimuli, such as driving or using potentially dangerous mechanical devices.

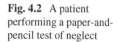

Fig. 4.2 A patient performing a paper-and-pencil test of neglect

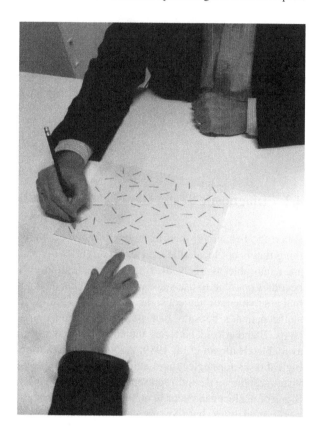

4.4   Visuo-perceptual Tests

Visuo-perceptual tests do not typically require substantial motor activity towards a certain sector of space; the patient has only to analyze a visual pattern and give a verbal response. In fact, although some of these tests require very little visuomotor activity, others require a substantial amount of active visual exploration, often with manual pointing directed to a defined portion of space.

4.4.1   Wundt–Jastrow Illusion

An example of visuo-perceptual tests is a lateralized version (Massironi et al. 1988) of the *Wundt–Jastrow illusion*. Two circular sectors, or fans, are presented one above the other. They are identical in area and shape, but when the longer curve of one fan is next to the shorter curve of the other, the first fan appears larger. However, neglect patients typically do not experience the illusion when the crucial part of the display appears on their left, neglected side (Fig. 4.3).

Fig. 4.3 The Wundt–Jastrow illusion modified by Massironi et al. (1988). The two fans have identical dimensions, but one is perceived as being longer (the lower ones in these examples). Neglect patients typically experience the illusion with the arrangement displayed in panel a, but not with the arrangement shown in panel b, where the crucial portion falls in the neglected left part of space (grayed circle)

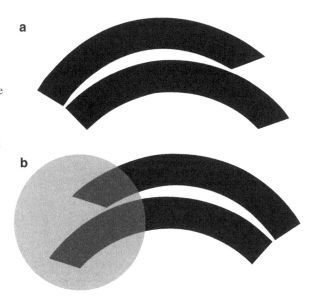

4.4.2 Overlapping Figures

Another test requiring little or no visuomotor activity is the *identification of overlapping figures*, presented in a limited area in central vision of the patient. This test was originally developed to assess disorders of visual recognition (Poppelreuter 1917) and has been used for neglect assessment by Gainotti and his co-workers (1971, 1986, 1991) (Fig. 4.4).

Patients typically omit naming the figures lying on the left part of the display. For patients with language disorders, a list containing the targets among distractor alternatives arranged in a vertical array can be presented below the test display. In this case, the patient is requested to point to the targets instead of naming them.

4.4.3 Search for Images

Relatively, more motor activity is required by the search for images or figures proposed by De Renzi et al. (1970), Chedru et al. (1973), and Gainotti et al. (1986) in large displays. Gainotti et al. (1986) have suggested that the manifestations of neglect are more specifically related to right hemisphere lesions for the first series of tasks but would be less lateralized when the task requires substantial visual exploration. These authors attributed this difference to the diverse nature of the collection of information carried in each series of tasks (more automatic in the first case, based on a partially intentional research activity in the second).

Fig. 4.4 An item from the Overlapping Figures Test (Gainotti et al. 1991). There are five displays (with a total of ten items) plus an initial training display. Participants have to name the lateralized figures or to point to them on a vertical multiple-choice array. Control participants usually do not omit more than one item on this test (Reproduced from Gainotti et al. (1991). © 1991, with permission from BMJ Publishing Group)

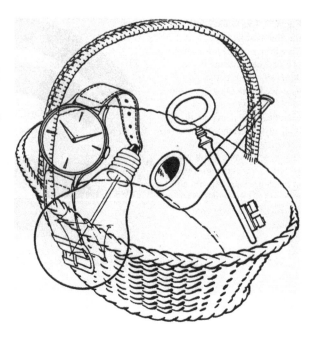

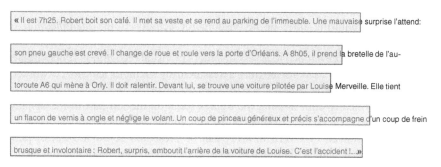

Fig. 4.5 Neglect dyslexia for sentences. This French patient neglected all the text shadowed in the figure and was able to read only the remaining portions on the extreme right-sided portion of the sheet

4.4.4   Reading in Neglect

Reading performance can be affected by visual neglect and can be evaluated by having patients read words, logatomes, or short phrases. During reading, neglect patients may omit the left part of words and sentences (so-called *neglect dyslexia*) (Fig. 4.5) (see Vallar et al. 2010, for review).

Reading often begins in the middle of the page, and line breaks are problematic, because the patient has trouble detecting the start of the new line in the left part of the page. In word reading, left-sided letters can be either omitted (deletion errors)

or replaced with other letters (substitution errors). This can result in choppy and inconsistent production, which curiously does not always seem to bother the patient (lack of awareness of the production errors is a general characteristic of neglect). Deletion errors are especially frequent when the right part of the word can have a meaning on its own (e.g., the compound word PASSPORT can be read "port"). Substitution errors often result in a word having approximately the same length as the target word (e.g., RIVER misread as "liver" or YELLOW as "pillow") (Ellis et al. 1987). Real words elicit fewer errors than logatomes (pronounceable non-words, such as YELVED), the so-called word superiority effect (Sieroff et al. 1988). For scoring purposes, neglect dyslexia errors are defined as errors in which target and error words are identical to the right of an identifiable *neglect point* in each word but have no letters in common to the left of the neglect point (Ellis et al. 1987). For example, the neglect point of YELLOW > "pillow" would be to the left of the first "l," but for YELLOW > "fellow" the neglect point would be to the left of the "e."

In rare cases, neglect dyslexia can be isolated, without other clinical signs of neglect (Costello and Warrington 1987). A study on 138 patients with acute/sub-acute (within 2 months) right hemisphere stroke (Lee et al. 2009) confirmed the possibility of dissociation of neglect dyslexia from other signs of neglect but also the rarity of an isolated neglect dyslexia. Signs of neglect dyslexia were present in 31 patients (23 %), while the frequency of neglect based on other neglect tasks was 58 % (80 patients). Of the 30 patients with neglect dyslexia, all but one had also other signs of neglect, which were often severe and associated to visual field defects. The most common lesion locations were centered on the TPJ but also combined with more ventral damage to the lingual and fusiform gyri.

4.5 Visuo-graphic Tests

The best known and most widely used tests of neglect involve the production of a graphic activity by the patient. Right-handed patients can usually perform these tests easily, because lesions in the right hemisphere do not impair movements with their preferred hand.

4.5.1 Drawing Tasks

Drawing tasks are usually quite easy to be performed and can be very informative. For these reasons, they are widely used in clinical evaluation.

Drawing can be performed either from memory (Fig. 4.6) or by copying a model. In the copy of drawings, the models can be simple geometric shapes (Arrigoni and De Renzi 1964; Gainotti 1968) or more spatially articulated figures, such as the schematic linear drawing of a landscape (Gainotti et al. 1972).

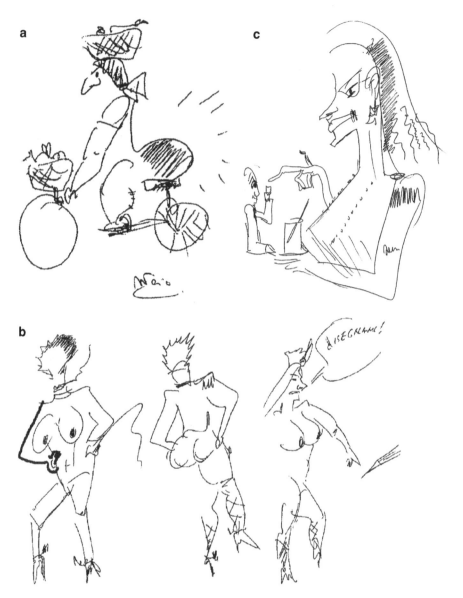

Fig. 4.6 (a–c) Spontaneous drawings made by Federico Fellini after a stroke in the right hemisphere. Note the omission of left details (Reproduced from Cantagallo and Della Sala (1998). © 1998, with permission from Elsevier)

The typical performance of neglect patients in drawing consists in omission or distortion of the details on the left side (Gainotti et al. 1972). Drawings often remain unfinished on the left side. Figure 4.6 displays spontaneous drawings made by the famous film director Federico Fellini, after he suffered from a stroke in the right hemisphere (Cantagallo and Della Sala 1998). As has been observed with other

Fig. 4.7 Daisy drawn from memory by a patient with left neglect. Note the left expansion with an increased number of left-sided petals (Reproduced from Rode et al. (2006). © 2006, with permission from Wolters Kluwer Health)

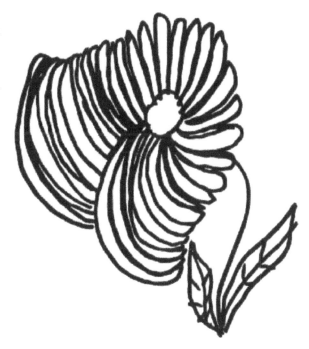

brilliant individuals (Dalla Barba et al. 1999; Bartolomeo 2013), Fellini retained partial insight into his condition and jokingly asked to include his new status of "neglector" in his calling card. However, he persisted in producing these drawings lacking left-side details. Thus, intellectual, or reflexive forms of consciousness (well preserved in the case of Fellini), may dissociate from more direct or immediate forms of consciousness, which are typically impaired in neglect patients (Bartolomeo and Dalla Barba 2002).

More rarely, left-sided distortions in drawing take the form of an expansion of the left portion of the patient's graphic production (Fig. 4.7). In the two right-brain-damaged patients described by Rode et al. (2006), left expansion occurred both in drawing from memory and by copying. The phenomenon did not depend on visual feedback, because it was present even when one patient was blindfolded. Nor did it depend on the direction of hand movements, because the same expansion occurred when patients performed the task through an epidiascope (where rightward hand movements are needed to reach the left part of the perceived scene).

4.5.1.1 Allochiria

Another rare but typical occurrence in drawing by copying is the displacement to the right side of the patients' copy of elements originally situated on the left side of the model (Halligan et al. 1992). These transposition errors are often referred to as *allochiria* or allesthesia. The last term is used by analogy with the behavior of

Fig. 4.8 Copy of drawings made by a patient with allochiria. Models (*left panel*) and patient's copies (*right panel*) of one- and two-winged butterflies. Note the transposition to the right of the round markings originally situated on the left-sided wing of the two-winged model butterfly (**c**) (Reproduced from Halligan et al. (1992). © 1992, with permission from BMJ Publishing Group Ltd.)

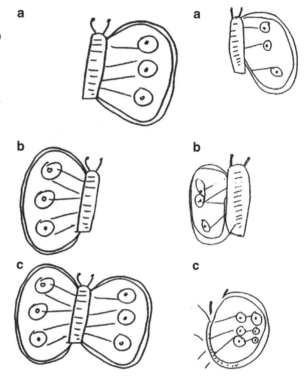

patients who report as occurring on the healthy side of their body a tactile stimulus given to the affected side (see Sect. 2.2). For example, a patient with a right fronto-parietal hemorrhage described by Halligan et al. (1992) sometimes omitted features and sometimes transposed them to the right side of the drawing. When copying a two-winged schematic butterfly, she omitted the left-sided wing and added corresponding features to the right-sided wing; however, one-winged butterflies were correctly copied irrespective of the side of occurrence of the wing in the model (Fig. 4.8).

Thus, it was only in the condition where a full butterfly was presented that transpositions took place. Another important consideration is that these patients fail to notice that their graphical production is inadequate to the model, despite the fact that the additions are located on the right, in principle the unaffected side of the drawing. This finding is consistent with several others which demonstrate that the "normal" right-sided space of neglect patients may actually not be normal at all.

4.5.1.2 Copy of Multielement Drawings: Scene-Based and Object-Based Neglect

When copying patterns composed of several elements aligned horizontally, some patients neglect the whole left part of the model, while others copy all the items but leave unfinished the left part of each (Gainotti et al. 1972; Marshall and Halligan

1993). These different patterns of performance have been respectively defined as scene- (or viewer-)based and object-based neglect (see Walker 1995, for review). Alternative terms for this dichotomy are egocentric and allocentric neglect, respectively. Figure 4.9 shows the performance of five different patients on the copy of a linear drawing of a landscape. Panels a–c demonstrate examples of scene-based neglect (with some object-based components indicated by the arrows); panel D shows an example of object-based neglect.

4.5.2 Cancellation Tasks

In cancellation tasks, patients are asked to cross out items scattered on a paper sheet such as lines (Albert 1973), letters (Mesulam 1985), or shapes (Gauthier et al. 1989; Halligan et al. 1991). Patients typically begin to scan the sheet from the right side, unlike normal left-to-right readers, who start from the left side (Bartolomeo et al. 1994). Patients omit a number of left-sided targets, sometimes without even reaching the midsection of the sheet (Fig. 4.10).

In the bells test (Gauthier et al. 1989) (Fig. 4.11), patients are requested to circle 35 targets (black ink drawings of bells), presented on a horizontal A4 paper sheet, along with 280 distractors. Targets and distractors are equally distributed in seven columns. Several scores can be calculated: the total number of omissions (out of the 35 responses), the difference between left-sided and right-sided omissions, and the participant's starting point (the column of the first circled target). The time taken to complete the task is also recorded. A total number of omissions superior to 6 are considered pathological, as well as a difference between left-sided and right-sided targets superior to 2 or an execution time longer than 183 s (Rousseaux et al. 2001).

In the similar letter cancellation task (Mesulam 1985), patients are presented with many letters disposed in a pseudorandom fashion and asked to cancel all the letters "A" (Fig. 4.12).

As noted by Gainotti et al. (2008), if line cancellation is a very easy test, cancellation of letters and shapes are much more demanding in terms of attentional selection because, in these tests, the target stimuli are mixed with distractors such as other letters or nontarget shapes. Studies that have compared the sensitivity of these various cancellation tests in neglect diagnosis showed that the demand in terms of attentional resources of a given test plays a role in the diagnostic sensitivity. The more selective attention is requested of the patient, the more numerous the left omissions (see Fig. 4.12). The general validity of this statement is confirmed by the fact that similar observations were made with very different tasks, such as those using Raven's colored matrices (Raven et al. 1976), whereby the patient must choose among central or lateralized alternatives the response that corresponds to the solution of a visuospatial problem. Even in this task, which is based on a visual-perceptual activity, the choice of alternatives ipsilateral to the cerebral lesion (a neglect index called "position preference" by Costa et al. 1969) increases gradually with increasing cognitive complexity (and therefore attentional load) of the task.

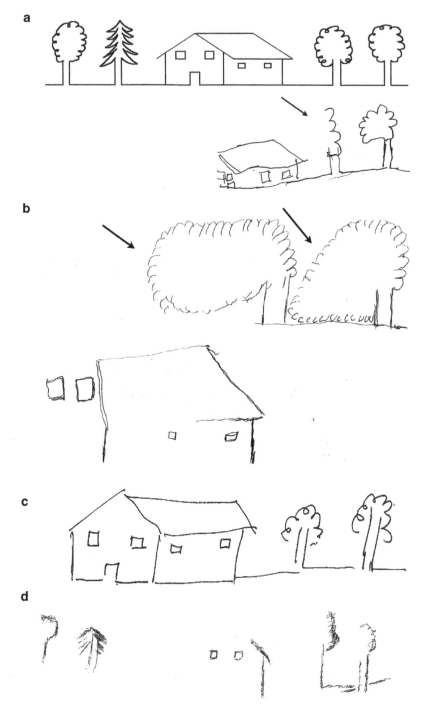

Fig. 4.9 Patterns of performance of different patients with left neglect on the landscape copy test. (**a**) Scene-based and object-based neglect (*arrow*). (**b**) Scene-based neglect with expansion of the left part of the trees (*arrows*). (**c**) Mild scene-based neglect (note the omitted baseline on the left of the house). (**d**) Object-based neglect

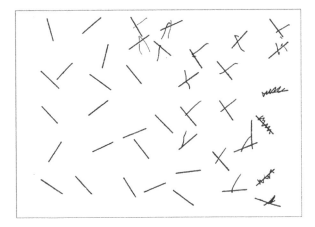

Fig. 4.10 Performance of a patient examined by Rode et al. (2007) on the line cancellation test (Albert 1973). Note how this patient not only neglected the left-sided targets but also was not able to reach the midsection of the bottom part of the sheet and kept cancelling again and again the right-sided lines (Reproduced from Rode et al. (2007), Fig. 10.1. © 2007, with permission from Oxford University Press)

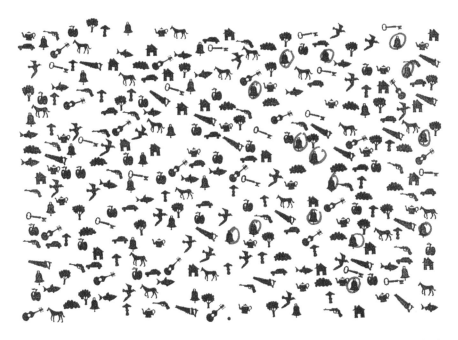

Fig. 4.11 Performance of a patient on the Bells test (Gauthier et al. 1989). The task is to circle all the bells present on the sheet

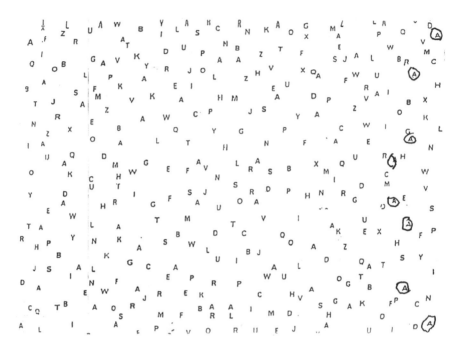

Fig. 4.12 Letter cancellation task. Note that this patient did not only omit targets on the left half of the sheet, she was able to find only the rightmost letters. Thus, neglect does not necessarily concern "the left half of space"; instead, the position of the left–right border can vary with the severity of neglect across patients (Marshall and Halligan 1989a), as well as with the difficulty of neglect tests

Patients' asymmetries of performance in cancellation tasks can vary from a few left-sided omissions to cancellation of only the rightmost items. Some patients will cancel again and again the same right-sided items, thus showing a pathological "revisiting behavior" for objects presented in the supposedly "normal" sector of space (Na et al. 1999; Rusconi et al. 2002; Mannan et al. 2005) (see Fig. 4.10).

This tendency either can result from perseverative deficits associated with prefrontal dysfunction or (perhaps depending on patients) can be influenced by patients' reactions to un-cancelled items within the neglected field. In support of the latter hypothesis, Manly et al. (2002) observed a progressive reduction of right-sided remarking behavior with decreasing numbers of left-sided (neglected) targets. In any case, right remarking strongly suggests that the putatively "normal" processing of right-sided items in these patients is not normal at all, because normal attention to these items would make patients cognizant of their previous markings of them.

Patients who can compensate for their deficit to some extent, as a result of either spontaneous recovery or after rehabilitation, may cancel out all the elements but keep starting from the right extremity of the sheet, at variance with normal participants, who most often start from the left part of the sheet (Bartolomeo et al. 1994), perhaps as a consequence of the left-to-right reading habits typical of Western

Fig. 4.13 Performance of a patient with left neglect on the bisection task. In this example, the lines are of different length and located in different positions on the left-right axis. Note the increasing rightward deviations with increasing line length. The first and last lines, placed in the left portion of the sheet, evoked an extreme midpoint deviation, repeated twice (*top line*) or even a complete neglect of the stimulus line (*bottom line*)

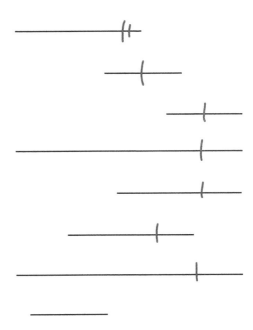

cultures (see Chokron et al. 1998). In one study on 206 right-brain-damaged patients (Azouvi et al. 2002), right starting on the Bells test was the single most sensitive sign of left neglect on paper-and-pencil tests.

4.5.3 Line Bisection

In line bisection tests, the patient is asked to mark with a pencil the center of a horizontal line in front of him or her. Neglect patients deviate the subjective midpoint to the right of the true center of the line (Fig. 4.13) (Colombo et al. 1976; Schenkenberg et al. 1980; Ishiai et al. 1989).

Several factors may influence the patterns of performance on line bisection, as described below.

4.5.3.1 Visual Field Defects

Visual field defects, such as left homonymous hemianopia (see Sect. 2.1), were once thought to cause neglect. Contrary to this hypothesis, there are patients with left hemianopia but no neglect, who deviate leftward on line bisection (Bartolomeo 1987; D'Erme et al. 1987; Barton and Black 1998). The association of left neglect and hemianopia, however, produces the largest rightward deviations on line bisection (Bartolomeo 1987; D'Erme et al. 1987; Doricchi and Angelelli 1999). When given relatively short lines to bisect (e.g., 5 cm or less), patients may paradoxically shift the bisection point leftwards, thus showing the so-called *crossover effect* (Marshall and Halligan 1989b). According to Doricchi and his co-workers, the copresence of visual field defects is a necessary condition for the crossover effect (Doricchi et al. 2005) and other neglect-related behaviors (Doricchi and Angelelli 1999) to occur. In the crossover effect, it has been suggested that patients with hom-onymous hemianopia or quadrantanopia might try to bring the left endpoint of the short line into the normal part of the visual field, thus deviating the subjective mid-dle towards that endpoint (Doricchi et al. 2005). Consistent with this hypothesis, a patient with left quadrantanopia showed a crossover effect only when the left end-point of the line was presented in his blind quadrant (Doricchi et al. 2003). For longer lines, whose right endpoint would occur well on the right in the patients' visual field, this mechanism would be offset by the concomitant attentional capture exerted by the right endpoint, which would then bias the patient's response towards the right (see Urbanski and Bartolomeo 2008). Actually, for longer lines the con-comitant presence of visual field defects (lateral homonymous hemianopia) is able to worsen the asymmetry of patients' performance, by shifting the bisection mark further rightward (Doricchi and Angelelli 1999).

4.5.3.2 Severity of Neglect

Koyama et al. (1997) administered line bisection to patients with moderate or severe neglect and observed two qualitatively distinct kinds of performance, depending on the severity of the disorder. In patients with mild or moderate neglect, the tendency to move rightward the subjective center of the line was influenced by the length and spatial position of the line. In contrast, in patients with severe neglect, these vari-ables did not influence patients' performance, which always tended to place the subjective center very close to the right end of the line. The first pattern of bisection was attributed by the authors to a lack of attention to the left half of the line (which could be influenced by characteristics of the visuospatial stimulus); on the other hand, severe neglect patients' performance was attributed to the attraction that the rightmost end of the stimulus automatically exerted on the patients' attention. These results are in good agreement with the hypothesis that several components can con-tribute to patients' performance in neglect, including decreased attention to stimuli located in the left half of the space and an automatic capture by those placed on the patient's right.

4.5.3.3 Position of the Line

The location in space of the line with respect to the patient's trunk midline also influences performance; rightward deviation increases when lines are located in the left hemispace and decreases when they are in the right hemispace (see Fig. 4.13) (Heilman and Valenstein 1979; Schenkenberg et al. 1980). This is a rather general phenomenon, which is observable with other neglect tests such as cancellation tasks.

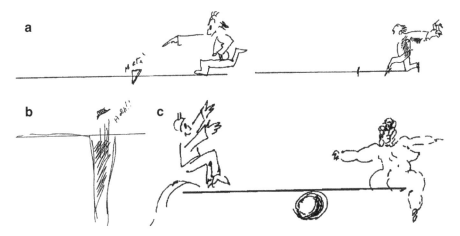

Fig. 4.14 (**a**) Lines bisected by Federico Fellini, who spontaneously added unrequested drawings (Cantagallo and Della Sala 1998). Here the graphic production suggests the typical right-to-left exploration pattern demonstrated by neglect patients. (**b**) Here, the pattern of exploration seems to go from the left to the right side, which is less common in neglect patients. However, the bisection mark (or, rather, the bisection drawing) remains displaced towards the right, perhaps because the weight of attention is on the right extremity of the line (**c**) (Reproduced from Cantagallo and Della Sala (1998). © 1998, with permission from Elsevier)

4.5.3.4   Patterns of Line Exploration

Another factor that influences line bisection performance is the direction of exploration of the line. Ishiai et al. (1989) monitored the patterns of eye fixation during line bisection and observed that, in contrast to hemianopic patients without neglect, patients with neglect and hemianopia never explored the left part of the line (in their blind field). Instead, they fixated a certain point on the right part of the line and marked the subjective midpoint there. Another patient with severe neglect (Ishiai et al. 1996) did explore the left part of the line, but his bisection points remained displaced rightward. The authors concluded that a rightward attentional bias was the predominant factor that determined where to place the subjective midpoint. Transient attentional shift to the left may produce leftward searches, but it does not induce effective processing of line bisection, perhaps because the "weight" of the patient's attention, or its tendency to be captured by right-sided objects, remains on the rightward extremity of the line (Urbanski and Bartolomeo 2008). An iconic representation of this hypothesis is provided by the humorous drawings that the famous film director Federico Fellini, who suffered from left neglect after a right hemisphere stroke (Cantagallo and Della Sala 1998), could not help adding to the right segments of his line bisections (Fig. 4.14).

Chokron et al. (1998) devised a passive version of line bisection, in which patients had to observe a dot or pen moving along the line and to say "stop" when it crossed the perceived middle. Neglect patients' rightward error decreased when the pen travelled from the left to the right, as opposed to the right-to-left condition, which increased the amount of rightward shift (Reuter-Lorenz and Posner 1990; Mattingley et al. 1994a; Urbanski and Bartolomeo 2008).

Reading habits seem also to influence line bisection, presumably through the induction of preferential exploratory strategies. Chokron and Imbert (1993) demonstrated that whereas left-to-right French readers deviated towards the left in a visuomotor line bisection task, right-to-left Israeli readers shifted the subjective middle towards the right.

4.5.3.5 Mechanisms of Subjective Center Shift in Line Bisection

A large body of evidence indicates that rightward deviation in line bisection cannot be completely explained by elementary sensory deficits (Fuchs 1920) or by deficits in programming hand movements towards the left side (Milner et al. 1993), although such problems may well contribute to patients' final performance (D'Erme et al. 1987; Bisiach et al. 1990; Doricchi and Angelelli 1999; Doricchi et al. 2005). According to Marshall and Halligan (1990), during line bisection neglect patients search the line for its midpoint from the right to the left and subsequently place the bisection point where the two hemi-segments appear to be of equal length. Evidence consistent with this hypothesis comes from the already mentioned eye-movement recordings, showing that neglect patients adopt a right-to-left scanning strategy and often fail to reach the leftmost extremity (Ishiai et al. 1989, 1992).

These notions are consistent with the possibility that an important component in rightward line bisection errors is an overestimation of the right portion of the line as compared to the left portion. This perceptual asymmetry might be related to a bias in attentional orienting, favoring rightward movements of attention, impairing leftward orienting, or both (see Bartolomeo and Chokron 2002, for review). Such an attentional bias might increase the perceptual salience of the right portion relative to the left portion of the line (Anderson 1996; Bultitude and Aimola Davies 2006). Thus, in line bisection the right and the left portion of the line would compete with each other until the point of subjective equality is reached. In left neglect, competition would be biased, causing the right portion to be overestimated with respect to the left portion. This, in turn, would bias the patients' response towards the right. The dysfunction of a right-hemisphere parietal–frontal network seems to be the lesional correlate of this biased competition (Doricchi and Tomaiuolo 2003; Thiebaut de Schotten et al. 2005; Bartolomeo 2006).

4.6   Representational (or Imaginal) Tasks

In his seminal paper on visuospatial deficits after right hemisphere damage, Russell Brain (1941) described a patient who, "when asked to describe how she would find her way from the tube station to her flat she described this in detail correctly and apparently visualizing the landmarks, but she consistently said right instead of left for the turning except on one occasion" (p. 259). When the patient reported by Denny-Brown et al. (1952) was asked to describe the hospital ward 2 months after

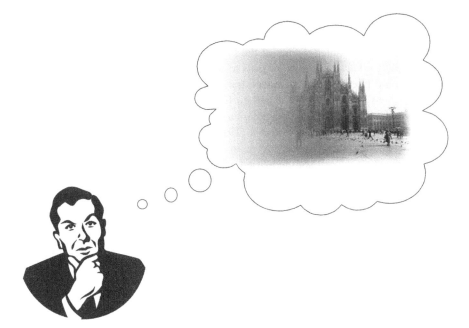

Fig. 4.15 In their seminal paper, Bisiach and Luzzatti (1978) reported two left neglect patients who, when asked to imagine and describe from memory familiar surroundings (the Piazza del Duomo in Milan), omitted mentioning left-sided details regardless of the imaginary vantage point that they chose, thus demonstrating imaginal/representational neglect (Figure as originally published in Bartolomeo et al. (2012))

being discharged, she "began by describing all the patients and the windows which had been on her right, mentioning them from right to left. She made no mention of the patients on the left until pressed and then was able to recall 2 out of 5" (Denny-Brown et al. 1952, p. 438–439).

Thus, patients with left spatial neglect may mention more right-sided than left-sided items when describing known places from memory. Bisiach and co-workers (1978, 1981) asked left neglect patients to imagine and describe familiar surroundings from memory (the Piazza del Duomo in Milan). Patients omitted mentioning left-sided details regardless of the imaginary vantage point that they assumed, thus showing representational, or imaginal, neglect (Fig. 4.15).

Bisiach and co-workers proposed that imaginal neglect could either result from "a representational map reduced to one half" (Bisiach et al. 1981) or from patients' failure to explore the left part of an intact map and preferred the amputation hypothesis on grounds of parsimony. The demonstration of imaginal neglect underlines the fact that unilateral neglect may not only occur during activities requiring the processing of sensory input but also during tasks less directly involved with perception, such as the description of places from memory. After their seminal paper (Bisiach and Luzzatti 1978), Bisiach and co-workers (1981) replicated this finding in a group study with 28 neglect patients, of which 13 were excluded from analysis because they misplaced the imagined details (e.g., they said that a left-sided detail was on the right side); the remaining 15 patients showed a bias towards mentioning more right-sided than left-sided details of the Piazza del Duomo. Bisiach, Luzzatti, and Perani (1979) asked 19 neglect patients to perform same/different judgments over pairs of cloud-like shapes that moved horizontally and could only be seen while passing behind a narrow slit, so that their form had to be mentally reconstructed to perform the task. Performance was particularly impaired when the shapes differed on the left side. Rode and co-workers (1995) reported eight neglect patients who gave poor descriptions of the left part of an imagined map of France. The number of items reported on the left side increased after vestibular stimulation of the left ear with cold water (Rode and Perenin 1994) (see Sect. 9.2.1). Grossi and his co-workers (1993) asked 24 neglect patients to judge the angle between imagined and seen clock hands. The ten patients who were able to complete the experiment made more errors when one of the hands was in the left hemispace, both in the imagery and in the perceptual condition.

Representational tasks are much less used clinically than classical visuo-perceptual or visuo-graphic tests. Even if tests of drawing objects from memory based on verbal instructions (a house, a clock, or a daisy) have long been used and offer a good diagnostic sensitivity in the detection of spatial neglect, these tests involve a substantial visuo-graphic component and therefore cannot make infer-ences about the level of impairment (visual or representational) in a particular patient (Chokron et al. 2004; Cristinzio et al. 2009). Imaginal neglect remains rela-tively less frequent than visual neglect (Bartolomeo et al. 1994, 2005) and has stim-ulated an important reflection on how to assess and demonstrate such a deficit and on the role of mental imagery in neglect (Beschin et al. 2000; Ortigue et al. 2001; Bartolomeo et al. 2005).

The tests used in the classical work of Bisiach et al. (1978, 1981) and in several subsequent investigations were based on the description from memory of places well known to the patients. These tests do not have any (explicit) perceptual com-ponents and thus enable the assessment of purely imaginal abilities. However, they pose other problems: (1) they do not lend themselves easily to a quantitative evalu-ation of imaginal neglect; (2) patients' familiarity with the place described varies from one subject to another and may also depend on patients' sociocultural environ-ment; and (3) the strategies used to solve this task can also vary. Thus, some patients, instead of maintaining the point of view that the examiner had asked them to adopt, seem, as it were, to "walk" along an imagined way. As a consequence, it becomes difficult to assess whether the described or forgotten buildings were actually on the right or on the left from the point of view of the patient. For this reason, other authors have adopted the different procedure of asking patients to imagine a map, presented in the standard view (i.e., with north to the top of the map), and to list all the cities they imagine "seeing" on this map (Rode and Perenin 1994; Bartolomeo et al. 2005). The description can then be repeated on an imagined upside-down map, with north at the bottom of the map. This procedure has the advantage of assessing imaginal neglect in a more quantitative and standardized way than place description.

Fig. 4.16 Geographical
locations mentioned by a
French patient with left
representational neglect on an
imagined map of France
(Rode et al. 2007). This map
shows the sequence of the
items (from 1 to 26)
mentioned by the patient
(Reproduced from Rode et al.
(2007), Fig. 10.1. © 2007,
with permission from Oxford
University Press)

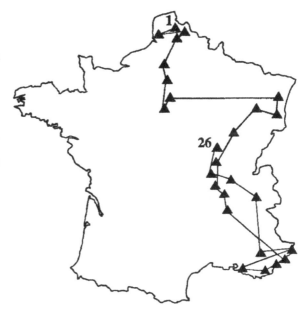

Rode and co-workers have exploited the wide and symmetrical geographical configuration of France by asking patients to imagine the map of France along the vertical axis that connects Perpignan to Lille and to state the largest number of geographical locations (towns, regions, etc.) that they imagine "seeing" on the right or on the left of this axis. Rode and his co-workers were able to confirm the existence of neglect in the left half of the imagined map (Fig. 4.16) and also to study the effect of various manipulations (such as vestibular stimulation and prism adaptation) on imaginal neglect (see Rode et al. 1995, for review). Importantly, when a patient with stable imaginal neglect had to list the towns of France without imagining them on a map, no asymmetry occurred (Rode et al. 2004). Thus, knowledge is preserved until the patient is asked to place it in space. The use of mental imagery, with an important spatial component in the case of an imagined map, is crucial to observe neglect-related asymmetries of performance.

4.6.1   Relation with Visual Tasks

In the above-reviewed group studies, imaginal neglect always co-occurred with visual neglect. However, single case reports have described both possible dissociations between visual and imaginal neglect: visual neglect in the absence of imaginal neglect (Anderson 1993; Coslett 1997) and imaginal neglect without visual neglect (Beschin et al. 1997; Coslett 1997; Guariglia et al. 1993). Also, a patient has been described who, after a left parieto-occipital hemorrhage and a right thalamic stroke, showed right visual neglect together with left imaginal neglect (Beschin et al. 2000).

To study the relationships between these two forms of neglect, Roman patients were asked to describe from memory three Roman piazzas, a map of Europe centered on Italy, and the Italian coast as it could be seen from the Sardinian coast (Bartolomeo et al. 1994). Thirty patients with right brain damage, 30 with left brain damage, and 30 normal individuals participated in the experiment. Seventeen patients with right brain damage and two left-brain-damaged patients had contralesional visual neglect. Imaginal neglect was present only in five right-brain-damaged patients, all showing signs of visual neglect. Thus, although imaginal neglect was always associated with visual neglect, the most frequent finding in right-brain-damaged patients was that of a visual neglect alone. The authors concluded in favor of an important role of right visual objects, as opposed to imagined scenes, in triggering neglect behavior, presumably because these objects attract patients' attention, which is typically biased rightward (see Sect. 6.1.1). In the study by Bartolomeo et al. (1994), there was no instance of imaginal neglect in isolation. However, such a dissociation was found when one of these patients with imaginal and visual neglect was followed up. Eight months after the first testing, this patient recovered from visual neglect, while imaginal neglect persisted longer. Later, another patient was identified who presented a similar pattern of selective recovery for visual, but not for imaginal, neglect (D'Erme et al. 1994 [abstract]). This patient did not show clinical signs of neglect 8 days after the stroke; he had, however, mild but definite left neglect signs on visuospatial testing and on imaginal tasks. Importantly, visual neglect at onset was so mild that it would probably have passed undetected without formal testing. Two weeks after the stroke, perceptual neglect had resolved, leaving an isolated representational neglect, which disappeared in turn 22 days after onset. Patient MN, described by Coslett (1997), also showed a similar pattern of selective recovery from perceptual, but not from representational, neglect (Coslett 1989 [abstract]).

Had these patients been tested only after recovery from visual neglect, they would have shown imaginal neglect in isolation. It is possible that these patients learned first to compensate for their neglect by exploring their visual space, which is more ecologically relevant and subject to feedback than mental images. Also, some techniques of neglect rehabilitation (see Chap. 9 below) may enhance leftward voluntary orienting of visual attention, thus reducing the perceptual but not the representational aspects of neglect (see Bartolomeo et al. 1994; Bartolomeo and Chokron 2001). Thus, patients may learn with time (and possibly the help of people around them) to compensate for their neglect in the visuospatial domain, but not in the more abstract imaginal domain, which is not the object of rehabilitation or of more informal reminders to "look at your left side."

Thus, imaginal neglect can double-dissociate from visual neglect, even if visual neglect in the absence of imaginal neglect seems to be a more frequent and perhaps more empirically robust pattern than the opposite dissociation (which could result from a difference in recovery rate rather than from a true difference in the underlying mechanisms). In the great majority of the cases reported in the literature, patients showed imaginal neglect for the left side of imagined scenes, as a result of a right hemisphere lesion (see, however, van Dijck et al. 2013, for a case of right imaginal neglect after left hemisphere damage). This pattern thus seems at sharp variance with other mental imagery deficits (such as those for object form and color or for orthographic material) which preferentially occur after left hemisphere lesions (with the possible exception of mental imagery of faces) (Bartolomeo 2002).

4.7   Other Spatial Sectors: "Near" and "Far" Neglect, Personal Neglect

Space is not a homogeneous medium for the brain. Extensive neurophysiologic and neuropsychological evidence indicate that neurocognitive processing of objects in space is different according to the sector of space involved: personal (bodily) space, extrapersonal space within reaching distance (peripersonal space), or extrapersonal space outside manual reaching (locomotor space) (Fig. 4.17). Interestingly, this division is not fixed, but can be dynamically remapped. For example, far space can be remapped as near space by the use of rigid tools, such as a rake to retrieve distant objects. This has been shown both in monkeys (Iriki et al. 1996) and in brain-damaged human patients with neglect (Berti et al. 2001).

4.7.1   Near vs. Far Space

The preceding sections essentially deal with the clinically most explored condition that of neglect in the extrapersonal space within reaching distance (near extrapersonal or peripersonal space). However, Brain (1941) had already suggested a

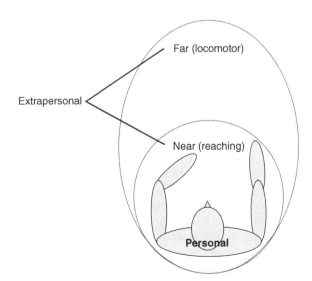

Fig. 4.17 Schematic representation of the sectors of space that can be selectively affected by neglect

distinction between the space at hand (reaching distance) and the space within walking distance. In the monkey, unilateral ablation of the FEF (area 8) produced more neglect for objects in contralesional far space than in near space; by contrast, unilateral ablation of frontal area 6, which receives direct projections from area 7b (the rostral part of the IPL), resulted in neglect in contralesional peripersonal (near) space (Rizzolatti et al. 1983). Drawing on this evidence, Halligan and Marshall (1991) described a human patient with severe neglect on conventional line bisection, but accurate performance with horizontal lines displayed at a distance of 2.44 m. The patient was able to correctly indicate the midpoint of these "far" lines either by using a projection light pen or by throwing darts. The opposite dissociation has also been reported (Cowey et al. 1994; Vuilleumier et al. 1998). However, another study (Pizzamiglio et al. 1989b) which employed a purely perceptual task such as the Wundt–Jastrow illusion (see Sect. 4.4.1), found no instance of near–far dissociation in a group of 70 right-brain-damaged patients. Thus, dissociations of performance concerning near and far stimuli might only occur with visuomotor tasks such as line bisection.

4.7.2   Personal Neglect

Neglect can also affect the space on the surface of the patient's body. Personal neglect, which shows obvious similarities with some of the disorders described in Chap. 3, can dissociate from extrapersonal neglect, although the occurrence of an isolated personal neglect is not common (Bisiach et al. 1986). The space around and inside the mouth can also be affected, with impaired swallowing, presence of food debris in the left hemibuccal space, and loss of saliva from the left side of the mouth (Andre et al. 2000). Personal neglect manifests itself as a lack of exploration of the contralesional part of the patients' body, to the extent that patients seem to "forget" the left part of their body during daily activities (bathing, dressing, shaving, or makeup) or fail to designate these body parts. Bisiach et al. (1986) devised a semi-quantitative test of personal neglect. Patients lie with their left arm positioned at the side of the trunk; the examiner, clearly pointing to the patient's right hand, says "With this hand, touch your other hand." A four-level scale was used for scoring: 0 (the patient promptly reaches for the target), 1 (the target is reached with hesitation and search), 2 (the search is interrupted before the target is reached), and 3 (no attempt to reach the target). This test is now part of the GEREN neglect battery (Azouvi et al. 2006). In the *comb and razor test*, patients may also be asked to comb their hair, shave, or put on makeup (Beschin and Robertson 1997; McIntosh et al. 2000). Another test requires the use of three objects (eyeglasses, a razor or powder, and a comb) in the body space (Zoccolotti and Judica 1991; Zoccolotti et al. 1992). For each object, scores are assigned, ranging from 0 to 3 on the basis of the asymmetry in performance of the patient in the left and right body space (0, no asymmetry; 3, maximal asymmetry). The final score consists of the sum of the evaluations obtained for each object, with an arbitrary cutoff of 2 (0–1=absence of personal neglect, 2–9=personal neglect from minor to severe) (Committeri et al. 2007). A more quantitative test is the *Fluff test* (Cocchini et al. 2001), which requires blindfolded patients to remove 24 2-cm diameter stickers attached with velcro to the front of their clothes. Fifteen of the stickers are placed on the left part of the body, 9 on the right part (Fig. 4.18).

Patients are not informed of the total number of targets. The number of removed stickers on the left and on the right part of the body is considered as a measure of the symmetry of patients' performance. None of the control participants of the study by Cocchini et al. (2001) omitted more than two left-sided stickers; thus a cutoff of 13 has been proposed for diagnosis of personal neglect.

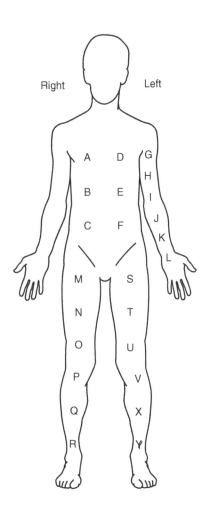

Fig. 4.18 Localization of the stickers in the Fluff test (Cocchini et al. 2001)

4.8   Ecological Assessment of Neglect

With time, neglect patients sometimes "learn" to perform the paper-and-pencil tasks reviewed above and may achieve normal performance on these tests. However, as soon as they exit the testing room, these patients may be seen bumping again into furniture on their left side and persist in neglecting objects in their everyday life. Thus, assessment of neglect by traditional neuropsychological tools may be insufficient to gather a complete picture of the pattern of deficits shown by an individual patient. Such dissociations may depend on the relative sparing of voluntary orienting mechanisms which may be involved in the overlearned, conventional tests, contrasting with an impairment of exogenous orienting (see Sect. 6.1.1), which results in attention being automatically captured by unexpected stimuli in everyday life (Seron et al. 1989). Thus, in addition to paper-and-pencil batteries, there is a need for standardized ecological measures of neglect to quantify the extent of neglect in everyday life, to adapt rehabilitation to the individual patient's limitations, to monitor changes, and to assess the effectiveness of rehabilitation (Azouvi et al. 2006). This last point is of great importance for rehabilitation studies, which are often limited by the lack of evidence of any therapeutic effect on everyday life skills (Robertson 1999; Bowen et al. 2002, 2013).

Several ecological assessment measures have been proposed in the literature (see Azouvi et al. 2006, for review), based either on the simulation of realistic conditions or on questionnaires attempting to measure patients' subjective account of everyday difficulties (Wilson et al. 1987; Towle and Lincoln 1991; Zoccolotti and Judica 1991). Towle and Lincoln (1991) proposed a questionnaire on neglect in everyday life, including 19 questions each with a dichotomous score. The questionnaire is filled out by the patient or a relative. The Behavioural Inattention Test (Wilson et al. 1987) includes nine behavioral subtests, based on the simulation of realistic conditions, such as reading a menu, a newspaper article, a road map, sorting coins, setting, or reading the time. Performance on these subtests correlated with a checklist score completed by an occupational therapist. This battery demonstrated good inter–rater and test–retest reliability. However, it did not seem to be more sensitive than paper-and-pencil tests. A semi-structured scale exploring personal and extrapersonal neglect was developed (Pizzamiglio et al. 1989a; Zoccolotti and Judica 1991; Zoccolotti et al. 1992). Extrapersonal neglect is assessed by asking patients to serve tea or to distribute cards to four persons around a square table and to describe complex figures and objects in a room. Personal neglect is explored by requiring the patient to use common objects (razor or powder, comb, glasses; see Sect. 4.7.2). There is good inter-rater reliability (Zoccolotti et al. 1992). Only extrapersonal subtests correlated with the results of paper-and-pencil tests. The comb and razor test is a modified version of the personal subscale with a more precise quantitative scoring system (Beschin and Robertson 1997; McIntosh et al. 2000). The Baking Tray Task consists of 16 wooden cubes that the patient is required to place as evenly as possible over a 75×100-cm board, "as if they were buns on a baking tray" (Tham and Tegner 1996). As expected, neglect patients tend to place the cubes preferentially on the right part of the board.

Azouvi et al. (2006) noted, however, that these tasks are all simulations of real-life situations, but they do not provide any direct and objective information on the patient's behavior in his actual everyday environment. Most of these ecological tests still represent quite artificial situations, which may rely more on voluntary rather than automatic orienting of attention. Moreover, they do not take into account anosognosia. On the basis of these considerations, another test battery was developed by the French-speaking neuropsychological community (GEREN), the "Batterie d'évaluation de la négligence spatiale" (Azouvi et al. 2002). This battery comprises two parts. The first part includes traditional clinical and "paper-and-pencil" tests of neglect and related disorders (such as extinction or visual field defects); the second part is a standardized observational scale, aimed at providing an ecological assessment of neglect in the patient's everyday life. The Catherine Bergego Scale is based on a direct observation of the patient's functioning in ten real-life situations, such as grooming, dressing, or wheelchair driving (Bergego et al. 1995). For each item, a four-point scale is used, ranging from 0 (no neglect) to 3 (severe neglect). To assess patients' awareness of neglect-related everyday difficulties, a parallel form of the scale has been designed as a questionnaire, with the same ten items previously described. An anosognosia score can be computed by recording the difference between the observer's and the patient's scores. There is good inter-rater reliability (Bergego et al. 1995) and, more importantly, the scale is able to detect signs of neglect in patients with normal performance on paper-and-pencil tests. For example, in a study on 69 unselected right-brain-damaged patients (Azouvi et al. 2002), six patients performed within the normal range on the Bells test, but nevertheless showed a moderate to severe behavioral neglect on the Catherine Bergego Scale. In the same study, patients' self-assessment was significantly lower than the examiners' score, indicating some form of anosognosia of neglect-related difficulties in everyday life. As suggested by Bowen et al. (2002), behavioral measures such as the Catherine Bergego Scale should be included in any therapeutic trial of neglect.

References

Albert ML. A simple test of visual neglect. Neurology. 1973;23:658–64.

Anderson B. Spared awareness for the left side of internal visual images in patients with left-sided extrapersonal neglect. Neurology. 1993;43:213–16.

Anderson B. A mathematical model of line bisection behaviour in neglect. Brain. 1996;119: 841–50.

Andrade K, Samri D, Sarazin M, Cruz De Souza L, Cohen L, Thiebaut de Schotten M, Dubois B, Bartolomeo P. Visual neglect in posterior cortical atrophy. BMC Neurol. 2010;10:68.

Andrade K, Kas A, Valabrègue R, Samri D, Sarazin M, Habert MO, Dubois B, Bartolomeo P. Visuospatial deficits in posterior cortical atrophy: structural and functional correlates. J Neurol Neurosurg Psychiatr. 2012;83:860–863.

Andre JM, Beis JM, Morin N, Paysant J. Buccal hemineglect. Arch Neurol. 2000;57:1734–41.

Arrigoni G, De Renzi E. Constructional apraxia and hemispheric locus of lesion. Cortex. 1964;1:180–97.

Azouvi P, Samuel C, Louis-Dreyfus A, Bernati T, Bartolomeo P, Beis J-M, Chokron S, Leclercq M, Marchal F, Martin Y, de Montety G, Olivier S, Perennou D, Pradat-Diehl P, Prairial C, Rode G, Sieroff E, Wiart L, Rousseaux M. Sensitivity of clinical and behavioural tests of spatial neglect after right hemisphere stroke. J Neurol Neurosurg Psychiatry. 2002;73:160–6.
Azouvi P, Bartolomeo P, Beis J-M, Perennou D, Pradat-Diehl P, Rousseaux M. A battery of tests for the quantitative assessment of unilateral neglect. Restor Neurol Neurosci. 2006;24:273–85.
Bartolomeo P. The novelty effect in recovered hemineglect. Cortex. 1997;33:323–32.
Bartolomeo P. The relationship between visual perception and visual mental imagery: a reappraisal of the neuropsychological evidence. Cortex. 2002;38:357–78.
Bartolomeo P. A parieto-frontal network for spatial awareness in the right hemisphere of the human brain. Arch Neurol. 2006;63:1238–41.
Bartolomeo P. The delusion of the master: the last days of Henry James. Neurol Sci. 2013;34(11): 2031–4.
Bartolomeo P. Aspetti dell'emi-inattenzione spaziale nelle lesioni emisferiche: fattori che influenzano la bisezione di linee [Aspects of spatial hemi-inattention: factors influencing line bisection performance]. In: Facoltà di Medicina. Unpublished M.D. thesis, Roma: Università Cattolica; 1987.
Bartolomeo P, Chokron S. Levels of impairment in unilateral neglect. In: Boller F, Grafman J, editors. Handbook of neuropsychology. 2nd ed. Amsterdam: Elsevier Science Publishers; 2001. p. 67–98.
Bartolomeo P, Chokron S. Orienting of attention in left unilateral neglect. Neurosci Biobehav Rev. 2002;26:217–34.
Bartolomeo P, Dalla Barba G. Varieties of consciousness (Commentary on Perruchet and Vinter: the self-organizing consciousness). Behav Brain Sci. 2002;25:331–2.
Bartolomeo P, D'Erme P, Gainotti G. The relationship between visuospatial and representational neglect. Neurology. 1994;44:1710–14.
Bartolomeo P, Dalla Barba G, Boissé MT, Bachoud-Lévi AC, Degos JD, Boller F. Right-side neglect in Alzheimer's disease. Neurology. 1998;51:1207–9.
Bartolomeo P, Urbanski M, Chokron S, Chainay H, Moroni C, Siéroff E, Belin C, Halligan P. Neglected attention in apparent spatial compression. Neuropsychologia. 2004;42:49–61.
Bartolomeo P, Bachoud-Lévi A-C, Azouvi P, Chokron S. Time to imagine space: a chronometric exploration of representational neglect. Neuropsychologia. 2005;43:1249–57.
Bartolomeo P, Thiebaut de Schotten M, Chica AB. Brain networks of visuospatial attention and their disruption in visual neglect. Front Hum Neurosci. 2012;6:110.
Barton JJ, Black SE. Line bisection in hemianopia. J Neurol Neurosurg Psychiatry. 1998;64: 660–2.
Beis JM, Keller C, Morin N, Bartolomeo P, Bernati T, Chokron S, Leclercq M, Louis-Dreyfus A, Marchal F, Martin Y, Perennou D, Pradat-Diehl P, Prairial C, Rode G, Rousseaux M, Samuel C, Sieroff E, Wiart L, Azouvi P. Right spatial neglect after left hemisphere stroke: qualitative and quantitative study. Neurology. 2004;63:1600–5.
Bergego C, Azouvi P, Samuel C, Marchal F, Louis-Dreyfus A, Jokic C, Morin L, Renard C, Pradat-Diehl P, Deloche G. Validation d'une échelle d'évaluation fonctionnelle de l'héminégligence dans la vie quotidienne: l'échelle CB. Ann Readapt Med Phys. 1995;38:183–9.
Berti A, Smania N, Allport A. Coding of far and near space in neglect patients. Neuroimage. 2001;14:S98–102.
Beschin N, Cocchini G, Della Sala S, Logie R. What the eyes perceive, the brain ignores: A case of pure unilateral representational neglect. Cortex. 1997;33:3–26.
Beschin N, Robertson IH. Personal versus extrapersonal neglect: a group study of their dissociation using a reliable clinical test. Cortex. 1997;33:379–84.
Beschin N, Basso A, Della Sala S. Perceiving left and imagining right: dissociation in neglect. Cortex. 2000;36:401–14.
Bisiach E, Luzzatti C. Unilateral neglect of representational space. Cortex. 1978;14:129–33.
Bisiach E, Luzzatti C, Perani D. Unilateral neglect, representational schema and consciousness. Brain. 1979;102:609–18.

Bisiach E, Capitani E, Luzzatti C, Perani D. Brain and conscious representation of outside reality. Neuropsychologia. 1981;19:543–51.

Bisiach E, Perani D, Vallar G, Berti A. Unilateral neglect: personal and extra-personal. Neuropsychologia. 1986;24:759–67.

Bisiach E, Geminiani G, Berti A, Rusconi ML. Perceptual and premotor factors of unilateral neglect. Neurology. 1990;40:1278–81.

Bonato M. Neglect and extinction depend greatly on task demands: a review. Front Hum Neurosci. 2012;6:195.

Bowen A, Lincoln NB, Dewey ME. Spatial neglect: is rehabilitation effective? Stroke. 2002;33:2728–9.

Bowen A, Hazelton C, Pollock A, Lincoln Nadina B. Cognitive rehabilitation for spatial neglect following stroke. In: Cochrane Database of Systematic Reviews: John Wiley & Sons, Ltd. 2013. doi:10.1002/14651858.CD003586.pub3.

Brain RW. Visual disorientation with special reference to lesion of the right brain hemisphere. Brain. 1941;64:244–72.

Bultitude JH, Aimola Davies AM. Putting attention on the line: investigating the activation-orientation hypothesis of pseudoneglect. Neuropsychologia. 2006;44:1849–58.

Cantagallo A, Della Sala S. Preserved insight in an artist with extrapersonal spatial neglect. Cortex. 1998;34:163–89.

Chedru F, Leblanc M, Lhermitte F. Visual searching in normal and brain-damaged subjects (contribution to the study of unilateral inattention). Cortex. 1973;9:94–111.

Chokron S, Imbert M. Influence of reading habits on line bisection. Cogn Brain Res. 1993;1:219–22.

Chokron S, Bartolomeo P, Perenin MT, Helft G, Imbert M. Scanning direction and line bisection: a study of normal subjects and unilateral neglect patients with opposite reading habits. Cogn Brain Res. 1998;7:173–8.

Chokron S, Colliot P, Bartolomeo P. The role of vision in spatial representation. Cortex. 2004;40:281–90.

Cocchini G, Beschin N, Jekhonen M. The fluff test: a simple task to assess body representation neglect. Neuropsychol Rehabil. 2001;11:17–31.

Colby CL, Goldberg ME. Space and attention in parietal cortex. Annu Rev Neurosci. 1999;22:319–49.

Colombo A, De Renzi E, Faglioni P. The occurrence of visual neglect in patients with unilateral cerebral disease. Cortex. 1976;12:221–31.

Committeri G, Pitzalis S, Galati G, Patria F, Pelle G, Sabatini U, Castriota-Scanderbeg A, Piccardi L, Guariglia C, Pizzamiglio L. Neural bases of personal and extrapersonal neglect in humans. Brain. 2007;130:431–41.

Coslett HB. Neglect in vision and visual imagery: a double dissociation. Brain. 1997;120:1163–71.

Coslett HB. Dissociation of attentional mechanisms in vision: evidence from neglect. J Clin Exp Neuropsychol. 1989;11:80 [abstract].

Costa LD, Vaughan Jr G, Horwitz M, Ritter W. Patterns of behavioral deficit associated with visual spatial neglect. Cortex. 1969;5:242–63.

Costello AD, Warrington EK. The dissociation of visuospatial neglect and neglect dyslexia. J Neurol Neurosurg Psychiatry. 1987;50:1110–16.

Cowey A, Small M, Ellis S. Left visuo-spatial neglect can be worse in far than in near space. Neuropsychologia. 1994;32:1059–66.

Cristinzio C, Bourlon C, Pradat-Diehl P, Trojano L, Grossi D, Chokron S, Bartolomeo P. Representational neglect in "invisible" drawing from memory. Cortex. 2009;45:313–17.

D'Erme P, De Bonis C, Gainotti G. Influenza dell'emi-inattenzione e dell'emianopsia sui compiti di bisezione di linee nei pazienti cerebrolesi [Influence of unilateral neglect and hemianopia on line bisection performance in brain-damaged patients]. Arch Psicol Neurol Psichiatr. 1987;48:165–89.

D'Erme P, Bartolomeo P, Gainotti G. Difference in recovering rate between visuospatial and representational neglect. Program and Abstracts, International Neuropsychological Society, 17th Annual European Conference. 1994;49.

Dalla Barba G, Bartolomeo P, Ergis AM, Boissé MF, Bachoud-Lévi AC. Awareness of anosognosia following head trauma. Neurocase. 1999;5:59–67.

De Renzi E, Faglioni P, Scotti G. Hemispheric contribution to the exploration of space through the visual and tactile modality. Cortex. 1970;6:191–203.

Denes G, Semenza C, Stoppa E, Lis A. Unilateral spatial neglect and recovery from hemiplegia: a follow-up study. Brain. 1982;105:543–52.

Denny-Brown D, Meyer JS, Horenstein S. The significance of perceptual rivalry resulting from parietal lesion. Brain. 1952;75:433–71.

Doricchi F, Angelelli P. Misrepresentation of horizontal space in left unilateral neglect: role of hemianopia. Neurology. 1999;52:1845–52.

Doricchi F, Tomaiuolo F. The anatomy of neglect without hemianopia: a key role for parietal-frontal disconnection? NeuroReport. 2003;14:2239–43.

Doricchi F, Guariglia P, Figliozzi F, Magnotti L, Gabriele G. Retinotopic modulation of space misrepresentation in unilateral neglect: evidence from quadrantanopia. J Neurol Neurosurg Psychiatry. 2003;74:116–19.

Doricchi F, Guariglia P, Figliozzi F, Silvetti M, Bruno G, Gasparini M. Causes of cross-over in unilateral neglect: between-group comparisons, within-patient dissociations and eye movements. Brain. 2005;128:1386–406.

Ellis AW, Flude BM, Young AW. "Neglect dyslexia" and the early visual processing of letters in words and nonwords. Cogn Neuropsychol. 1987;4:439–64.

Fuchs W. Untersuchung über das Sehen der Hemianopiker und Hemiamblyopiker. Z Psychol Physiol Sinnersorg. 1920;84:67–169.

Gainotti G. Les manifestations de négligence et d'inattention pour l'hémi-espace. Cortex. 1968;4:64–91.

Gainotti G. The role of automatic orienting of attention towards ipsilesional stimuli in non-visual (tactile and auditory) neglect: a critical review. Cortex. 2010;46:150–60.

Gainotti G, Tiacci C. The relationships between disorders of visual perception and unilateral spatial neglect. Neuropsychologia. 1971;9:451–458.

Gainotti G, Messerli P, Tissot R. Qualitative analysis of unilateral spatial neglect in relation to the laterality of cerebral lesions. J Neurol Neurosurg Psychiatry. 1972;35:545–50.

Gainotti G, D'Erme P, Monteleone D, Silveri MC. Mechanisms of unilateral spatial neglect in relation to laterality of cerebral lesions. Brain. 1986;109:599–612.

Gainotti G, D'Erme P, Bartolomeo P. Early orientation of attention toward the half space ipsilateral to the lesion in patients with unilateral brain damage. J Neurol Neurosurg Psychiatry. 1991;54:1082–9.

Gainotti G, Bourlon C, Bartolomeo P. La négligence spatiale unilatérale. In: Lechevalier B, Viader F, Eustache F, editors. Traité de neuropsychologie clinique. Bruxelles/Paris: De Boeck/INSERM; 2008. p. 627–49.

Gauthier L, Dehaut F, Joanette Y. The bells test: a quantitative and qualitative test for visual neglect. Int J Clin Neuropsychol. 1989;11:49–53.

Grossi D, Angelini R, Pecchinenda A, Pizzamiglio L. Left imaginal neglect in heminattention: experimental study with the O'clock Test. Behavioural Neurology. 1993;6:155–58.

Guariglia C, Padovani A, Pantano P, Pizzamiglio L. Unilateral neglect restricted to visual imagery. Nature. 1993;364:235–7.

Halligan PW, Marshall JC. Left neglect for near but not far space in man. Nature. 1991;350:498–500.

Halligan PW, Marshall JC, Wade DT. Visuospatial neglect: underlying factors and test sensitivity. Lancet. 1989;334:908–12.

Halligan PW, Cockburn J, Wilson B. The behavioural assessment of visual neglect. Neuropsychol Rehabil. 1991;1:5–32.

Halligan PW, Marshall JC, Wade DT. Left on the right: allochiria in a case of left visuo-spatial neglect. J Neurol Neurosurg Psychiatry. 1992;55:717–19.

Heilman KM, Valenstein E. Mechanisms underlying hemispatial neglect. Ann Neurol. 1979;5:166–70.

Hughlings Jackson J. Case of large cerebral tumour without optic neuritis and with left hemiplegia and imperception. In: Taylor J, editors. Selected writings of John Hughlings Jackson. London: Hodden and Stoughton; 1876/1932. p. 146–52.

Iriki A, Tanaka M, Iwamura Y. Coding of modified body schema during tool use by macaque postcentral neurones. NeuroReport. 1996;7:2325–30.

Ishiai S, Furukawa T, Tsukagoshi H. Visuospatial processes of line bisection and the mechanisms underlying unilateral spatial neglect. Brain. 1989;112:1485–502.

Ishiai S, Sugishita M, Mitani K, Ishizawa M. Leftward search in left unilateral spatial neglect. J Neurol Neurosurg Psychiatry. 1992;55:40–4.

Ishiai S, Seki K, Koyama Y, Gono S. Ineffective leftward search in line bisection and mechanisms of left unilateral spatial neglect. J Neurol. 1996;243:381–7.

Koyama Y, Ishiai S, Seki K, Nakayama T. Distinct processes in line bisection according to severity of left unilateral spatial neglect. Brain Cogn. 1997;35:271–81.

Lee BH, Suh MK, Kim EJ, Seo SW, Choi KM, Kim GM, Chung CS, Heilman KM, Na DL. Neglect dyslexia: frequency, association with other hemispatial neglects, and lesion localization. Neuropsychologia. 2009;47:704–10.

Manly T, Woldt K, Watson P, Warburton E. Is motor perseveration in unilateral neglect 'driven' by the presence of neglected left-sided stimuli? Neuropsychologia. 2002;40:1794–803.

Mannan SK, Mort DJ, Hodgson TL, Driver J, Kennard C, Husain M. Revisiting previously searched locations in visual neglect: role of right parietal and frontal lesions in misjudging old locations as new. J Cogn Neurosci. 2005;17:340–54.

Marshall JC, Halligan PW. Does the midsagittal plane play any privileged role in "left" neglect? Cogn Neuropsychol. 1989a;6:403–22.

Marshall JC, Halligan PW. When right goes left: an investigation of line bisection in a case of visual neglect. Cortex. 1989b;25:503–15.

Marshall JC, Halligan PW. Line bisection in a case of visual neglect: psychophysical studies with implications of theory. Cogn Neuropsychol. 1990;7:107–30.

Marshall JC, Halligan PW. Visuo-spatial neglect: a new copying test to assess perceptual parsing. J Neurol. 1993;240:37–40.

Massironi M, Antonucci G, Pizzamiglio L, Vitale MV, Zoccolotti P. The Wundt-Jastrow illusion in the study of spatial hemi-inattention. Neuropsychologia. 1988;26:161–6.

Mattingley JB, Bradshaw JL, Bradshaw JA. Horizontal visual motion modulates focal attention in left unilateral spatial neglect. J Neurol Neurosurg Psychiatry. 1994a;57:1228–35.

Mattingley JB, Bradshaw JL, Bradshaw JA, Nettleton NC. Residual rightward attentional bias after apparent recovery from right hemisphere damage: implications for a multicomponent model of neglect. J Neurol Neurosurg Psychiatry. 1994b;57:597–604.

McIntosh RD, Brodie EE, Beschin N, Robertson IH. Improving the clinical diagnosis of personal neglect: a reformulated comb and razor test. Cortex. 2000;36:289–92.

Mesulam MM. Attention, confusional states and neglect. In: Mesulam MM, editor. Principles of behavioral neurology. Philadelphia: F.A. Davis; 1985. p. 125–68.

Milner AD, Harvey M, Roberts RC, Forster SV. Line bisection errors in visual neglect: misguided action or size distortion? Neuropsychologia. 1993;31:39–49.

Na DL, Adair JC, Kang Y, Chung CS, Lee KH, Heilman KM. Motor perseverative behavior on a line cancellation task. Neurology. 1999;52:1569–76.

Nicklason F, Finucane P. "Hanging spectacles" sign in stroke. Lancet. 1990;336:1380.

Ortigue S, Viaud-Delmon I, Annoni JM, Landis T, Michel C, Blanke O, Vuilleumier P, Mayer E. Pure representational neglect after right thalamic lesion. Ann Neurol. 2001;50:401–4.

Perennou D. Postural disorders and spatial neglect in stroke patients: a strong association. Restor Neurol Neurosci. 2006;24:319–34.

Pizzamiglio L, Cappa S, Vallar G, Zoccolotti P, Bottini G, Ciurli P, Guariglia C, Antonucci G. Visual neglect for far and near extra-personal space in humans. Cortex. 1989a;25:471–7.

Pizzamiglio L, Judica A, Razzano C, Zoccolotti P. Toward a comprehensive diagnosis of visuo-spatial disorders in unilateral brain damaged patients. Psychol Assess. 1989b;5:199–218.

Poppelreuter W. Die psychischen Schädigungen durch Kopfschuss im Kriege 1914–1916. Leipzig: Voss; 1917.

Raven JC, Court JH, Raven J. Manual for Raven's progressive matrices. London: H.K. Lewis; 1976.

Reuter-Lorenz PA, Posner MI. Components of neglect from right-hemisphere damage: an analysis of line bisection. Neuropsychologia. 1990;28:327–33.

Rizzolatti G, Matelli M, Pavesi G. Deficits in attention and movement following the removal of postarcuate (area 6) and prearcuate (area 8) cortex in macaque monkeys. Brain. 1983;106 (Pt 3):655–73.

Robertson IH. Cognitive rehabilitation: attention and neglect. Trends Cogn Sci. 1999;3:385–93.

Robertson IH. Do we need the "lateral" in unilateral neglect? Spatially nonselective attention deficits in unilateral neglect and their implications for rehabilitation. Neuroimage. 2001;14: S85–90.

Rode G, Perenin MT. Temporary remission of representational hemineglect through vestibular stimulation. NeuroReport. 1994;5:869–72.

Rode G, Perenin MT, Boisson D. Négligence de l'espace représenté : mise en évidence par l'évocation mentale de la carte de France [Neglect of the representational space: demonstration by mental evocation of the map of France]. Rev Neurol. 1995;151:161–4.

Rode G, Rossetti Y, Perenin MT, Boisson D. Geographic information has to be spatialized to be neglected: a representational neglect case. Cortex. 2004;40:391–7.

Rode G, Michel C, Rossetti Y, Boisson D, Vallar G. Left size distortion (hyperschematia) after right brain damage. Neurology. 2006;67:1801–8.

Rode G, Luaute J, Klos T, Courtois-Jacquin S, Revol P, Pisella L, Holmes NP, Boisson D, Rossetti Y. Bottom-up visuo-manual adaptation: consequences for spatial cognition. In: Haggard P, Rossetti Y, Kawato M, editors. Attention and performance XXII: sensorimotor foundations of higher cognition. Oxford: Oxford University Press; 2007. p. 207–29.

Rousseaux M, Beis JM, Pradat-Diehl P, Martin Y, Bartolomeo P, Chokron S, Leclercq M, Louis-Dreyfus A, Marchal F, Pérénnou D, Prairial C, Samuel C, Siéroff E, Wiart L, Azouvi P. Normalisation d'une batterie de dépistage de la négligence spatiale. Etude de l'effet de l'âge, du niveau d'éducation, du sexe, de la main et de la latéralité [Presenting a battery for assessing spatial neglect. Norms and effects of age, educational level, sex, hand and laterality]. Rev Neurol. 2001;157:1385–401.

Rusconi ML, Maravita A, Bottini G, Vallar G. Is the intact side really intact? Perseverative responses in patients with unilateral neglect: a productive manifestation. Neuropsychologia. 2002;40:594–604.

Schenkenberg T, Bradford DC, Ajax ET. Line bisection and unilateral visual neglect in patients with neurologic impairment. Neurology. 1980;30:509–17.

Seron X, Deloche G, Coyette F. A retrospective analysis of a single case neglect therapy: a point of theory. In: Seron X, Deloche G, editors. Cognitive approaches in neuropsychological rehabilitation. Hillsdale: Lawrence Erlbaum Associates; 1989. p. 289–316.

Sieroff E, Pollatsek A, Posner MI. Recognition of visual letter strings following injury to the posterior visual spatial attention system. Cogn Neuropsychol. 1988;5:427–49.

Tham K, Tegner R. The baking tray task: a test of spatial neglect. Neuropsychol Rehabil. 1996;6:19–25.

Thiebaut de Schotten M, Urbanski M, Duffau H, Volle E, Levy R, Dubois B, Bartolomeo P. Direct evidence for a parietal-frontal pathway subserving spatial awareness in humans. Science. 2005;309:2226–8.

Towle D, Lincoln NB. Development of a questionnaire for detecting everyday problems in stroke patients with unilateral visual neglect. Clin Rehabil. 1991;5:135–40.

Urbanski M, Bartolomeo P. Line bisection in left neglect: the importance of starting right. Cortex. 2008;44:782–93.

Vallar G, Perani D. The anatomy of unilateral neglect after right-hemisphere stroke lesions. A clinical/CT-scan correlation study in man. Neuropsychologia. 1986;24:609–22.

Vallar G, Burani C, Arduino LS. Neglect dyslexia: a review of the neuropsychological literature. Exp Brain Res. 2010;206:219–35.

van Dijck JP, Gevers W, Lafosse C, Fias W. Right-sided representational neglect after left brain damage in a case without visuospatial working memory deficits. Cortex. 2013;49(9):2283–93.

Vuilleumier P, Valenza N, Mayer E, Reverdin A, Landis T. Near and far visual space in unilateral neglect. Ann Neurol. 1998;43:406–10.

Walker R. Spatial and object-based neglect. Neurocase. 1995;1:371–83.

Weintraub S, Mesulam MM. Visual hemispatial inattention: stimulus parameters and exploratory strategies. J Neurol Neurosurg Psychiatry. 1988;51:1481–8.

Weintraub S, Daffner KR, Ahern GL, Price BH, Mesulam MM. Right sided hemispatial neglect and bilateral cerebral lesions. J Neurol Neurosurg Psychiatry. 1996;60:342–4.

Wilson B, Cockburn J, Halligan P. Development of a behavioral test of visuospatial neglect. Arch Phys Med Rehabil. 1987;68:98–102.

Zoccolotti P, Judica A. Functional evaluation of hemineglect by means of a semistructured scale: personal extrapersonal differentiation. Neuropsychol Rehabil. 1991;1:33–44.

Zoccolotti P, Antonucci G, Judica A. Psychometric characteristics of two semi-structured scales for the functional evaluation of hemi-inattention in extrapersonal and personal space. Neuropsychol Rehabil. 1992;2:179–91.

Further Reading

Azouvi P, Olivier S, de Montety G, Samuel C, Louis-Dreyfus A, Tesio L. Behavioral assessment of unilateral neglect: study of the psychometric properties of the Catherine Bergego Scale. Arch Phys Med Rehabil. 2003;84(1):51–7.

Azouvi P, Bartolomeo P, Beis J-M, Perennou D, Pradat-Diehl P, Rousseaux M. A battery of tests for the quantitative assessment of unilateral neglect. Restor Neurol Neurosci. 2006;24: 273–85.

De Renzi E. Disorders of space elaboration and cognition. New York: Wiley; 1982.

Gainotti G, Bourlon C, Bartolomeo P. La négligence spatiale unilatérale. In: Lechevalier B, Viader F, Eustache F, editors. Traité de neuropsychologie clinique. Bruxelles/Paris: De Boeck/ INSERM; 2008. p. 627–49.

Parton A, Malhotra P, Husain M. Hemispatial neglect. J Neurol Neurosurg Psychiatry. 2004;75(1):13–21.

Robertson IH, Halligan P. Spatial neglect: a clinical handbook for diagnosis and treatment. Hove: Psychology Press; 1999.

Wilson B, Cockburn J, Halligan P. Development of a behavioral test of visuospatial neglect. Arch Phys Med Rehabil. 1987;68:98–102.

Chapter 5
Experimental Variants of Neglect Tests

Keywords Drawing • Cancellation • Line bisection • Representational tasks

5.1 Variants of Drawing Tasks: Blind Drawing

An important issue in drawing, as well as in neglect in general, concerns the role of visual feedback. Drawing tasks are sometimes considered active tasks, whereby attention, perception, and spatial exploration are restricted to the examination of the model to be drawn and virtually absent when the model is not there, as in drawing from memory. However, even in drawing from memory, perception of one's own graphic production can substantially influence the final outcome. For example, Chokron et al. (2004) asked neglect patients to draw common objects from memory both with their eyes open and while blindfolded. The results showed that some of these patients showed less neglect without visual input than with it (Fig. 5.1), thus confirming previous similar findings (Mesulam 1985; Anderson 1993). Chokron et al. explained their results in terms of an attentional bias, consisting in a "magnetic" capture of attention by the right-sided visual details the patient had just drawn (see above and Gainotti et al. 1991), which was obviously absent when visual details were suppressed by blindfolding. These findings caution against the direct use of drawing from memory to infer the status of mental representations (Bartolomeo 2002).

A similar conclusion was reached by Mark et al. (1988), who used variants of a cancellation task. As detailed in the following Sect. 5.2.1, in this study ten patients with left neglect erased lines or drew over them with a pencil mark. There was less neglect in the "erase" than in the "draw" condition. Mark et al. concluded that right-sided lines attracted patients' attention when they were crossed by a pencil mark, whereas rendering these lines invisible by erasing them obviously nullified this effect, thus decreasing neglect.

P. Bartolomeo, *Attention Disorders After Right Brain Damage*,
DOI 10.1007/978-1-4471-5649-9_5, © Springer-Verlag London 2014

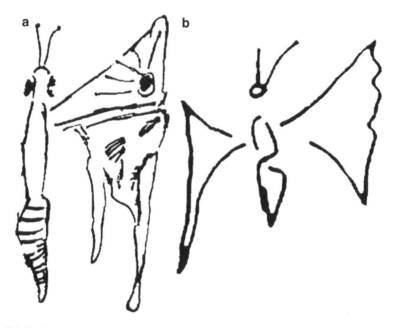

Fig. 5.1 Performance of a patient when drawing a butterfly from memory, with (**a**) and then without (**b**) visual guidance (while blindfolded), whereupon left neglect disappeared (Reproduced from Chokron et al. (2004). © 2004, with permission from Elsevier)

However, findings apparently conflicting with this account were reported in another cancellation study (Wojciulik et al. 2004), where more items were cancelled using visible marks than when using invisible marks (a pen with the cap on), perhaps because in the absence of visual markers, patients failed to remember which locations they had already visited (see Sect. 6.4.1). If so, then some patients might show more neglect without visual feedback even when drawing from memory, than with such feedback. Such a pattern of performance case was indeed described by Cristinzio et al. (2009). Their patient AG was requested to draw six items from memory with or without visual control. The items were a spider, a carafe, a butterfly, a pair of trousers, a sun, and an umbrella. To decrease the difficulty of drawing without visual feedback and to eliminate only visual and not visuomotor feedback, Cristinzio et al. added a further condition inspired by the Wojciulik et al.'s (2004) study, namely, drawing with the eyes open but using a pen with the cap on, so that the drawing was visible only via carbon paper. Thus, the task consisted of three conditions: (1) drawing with eyes open, (2) drawing with eyes open but using a pen with the cap on, and (3) drawing while blindfolded. Results showed that, in the absence of visual feedback (whether using carbon paper or blindfolding), patient AG systematically failed to draw more left-sided elements as compared to the condition with visual feedback (Fig. 5.2).

Fig. 5.2 Patient AG's rendition of a butterfly (*left*) and of a sun (*right*). In this patient, left neglect seemed enhanced by the absence of visual feedback (Reproduced from Cristinzio et al. (2009). © 2009, with permission from Elsevier)

Visual feedback

Carbon paper

Blindfolding

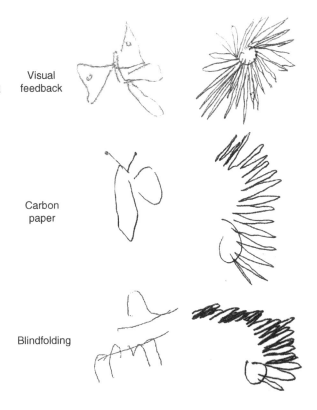

Thus, when drawing common objects from memory with or without visual feedback, patient AG demonstrated less neglect in the visual feedback condition. This contrasts with the performance of the patients reported by Chokron et al. (2004), who showed the opposite pattern of results, namely, more neglect with visual feedback than without. A possibility to explain this discrepancy is that these patients had different deficits, with preponderance of right attentional capture for the Chokron et al. patients and of a left representational impairment for the Cristinzio et al.'s patient. However, an account exclusively based on a representational impairment in AG leaves unexplained the decrease of neglect with visual feedback in this patient. A lateralized impairment of a mental representation of space (see Sect. 4.6) should influence drawing performance independently of the presence or absence of visual feedback.

Another way to explain the decrease of neglect with visual feedback in patient AG is to invoke the additional contribution to performance of a deficit of spatial working memory (see Sect. 6.4.1). According to this hypothesis, in the absence of visual feedback, AG was more likely to forget what he had already drawn and to perseverate in making (invisible) pen strokes on the right, ipsilesional side. Unfortunately, spatial working memory was not formally assessed in this patient, so this account remains speculative.

5.2   Variants of Cancellation Tasks

5.2.1   Erasing Targets

As mentioned before, Mark et al. (1988) used a different version of a cancellation task in order to test the hypothesis that a component of neglect for stimuli located on the left results from attraction exerted by right-sided items on the patient's spatial attention (see Sect. 6.1.1). To this end, Mark et al. (1988) administered to left neglect patients two different versions of a line cancellation test. In a control version lines were, as usual, crossed out with a pen stroke; in the experimental version, they were rather to be physically wiped out with an eraser. Since in each case the patients began by marking stimuli located on the right and then proceeded to the left, the crossed stimuli remained on the right (thus presumably attracting patients' attention) in the standard version of the test, while in the experimental version stimuli disappeared and consequently could not attract the patients' attention. Consistent with the hypothesis, the number of left omissions significantly decreased when the stimuli located on the right had been erased and could no longer automatically draw the patient's attention.

Another notable variant of cancellation tasks is the addition of a monetary reward for each cancelled item. This simple modification led to an increased exploration of the left part of the sheet, with consequent dramatic reduction of neglect (Mesulam 1985; Malhotra et al. 2013). This finding underlies the importance of motivational factors in neglect behavior and the possibility of circumventing neglect by manipulating task conditions apparently unrelated to space.

5.2.2   "Invisible" Cancellation Marks

As mentioned in Sect. 5.1, Wojciulik et al. (2004) hypothesized the presence of a nonlateralized deficit in spatial working memory to account for the performance of a sample of neglect patients on a modified cancellation test (see Sect. 6.4.1). Similar to the "blind" drawing experiments described in Sect. 5.1, patients marked each target using either a normal pen or a pen with the cap on, so that the markings were invisible. Patients cancelled more items with visible than with invisible marks. Thus, visual feedback improved patients' performance. Wojciulik et al. (2004) concluded that failure to cancel the left items on the contralateral side in the condition employing invisible marks was due to a deficit of spatial working memory. Spatial working memory was indeed presumably required to keep track of previously found items only when marked invisibly (see also Husain et al. 2001, and Sect. 6.4). When present, such deficits can thus exacerbate left neglect on visual search tasks (Malhotra et al. 2005).

Fig. 5.3 Two different patterns of performance on the Ota et al.'s (2001) cancellation task. Patients were requested to mark with a cross the incomplete targets and to circle the complete ones. The *top panel* shows the performance of a patient with viewer-centered (or egocentric) neglect, who failed to mark targets on the left side of the display. The *lower panel* shows the performance of a patient with stimulus- or object-centered or allocentric neglect, who incorrectly marked stimuli with left gaps as complete by circling them, whether they were on the left or the right side of the sheet (Reproduced from Khurshid et al. (2012). © 2012, with permission from Elsevier)

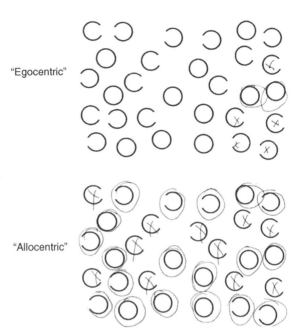

"Egocentric"

"Allocentric"

5.2.3   Left–Right Asymmetric Targets

Ota et al. (2001) devised a cancellation task apt to discriminate between scene-based and object-based neglect (see Sects. 4.5.1 and 6.1.4). In this task, targets are circles with an opening either on the left or on the right side and which are inter-mixed with full circle distractors. Patients are requested to mark all the open circles. Patients with scene-based (or egocentric) neglect omit the targets situated on the left part of the sheet, independent of the side of the gap (Fig. 5.3, top panel); patients with object-based (or allocentric) neglect fail to detect the left gaps no matter where these open circles are located on the sheet and may thus omit left-opened circles throughout the visual scene (bottom panel in Fig. 5.3).

5.3   Variants of Line Bisection

5.3.1   The Landmark Task

Instead of having patients mark with a pencil stroke the perceived center of horizontal lines, in the *landmark task* (Harvey et al. 1995) patients are presented with pre-bisected lines and are requested to judge whether the bisection mark is at

Fig. 5.4 Three example items of the landmark task (Milner et al. 1993). Item (**a**) is correctly bisected at its center, whereas the bisection tract is shifted to the right for item (**b**) and to the left for item (**c**). Patients have to establish whether the bisection mark is shifted towards the left or towards the right. Patients with left neglect might state that the correctly bisected item (**a**) has a left-deviated mark

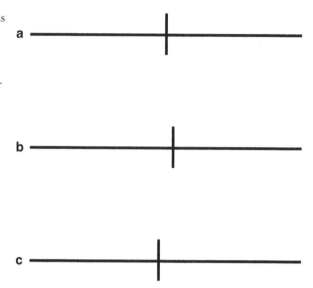

the center or not (Fig. 5.4). In this task, no manual action is required, at variance with classical line bisection. However, neglect patients typically reproduce their bisection behavior and consider the right segment as being longer than the left one (Milner et al. 1993). For example, they may state that the bisection mark on a correctly bisected line is shifted towards the left or that the left endpoint is closer to the center than the right endpoint.

5.3.2   Pseudoneglect and the Attentional Repulsion Effect

When neurologically healthy individuals bisect horizontal lines, they often make errors (much smaller than those of neglect patients) in the opposite direction and mark the bisection point to the *left* of the true center, a phenomenon dubbed "pseudoneglect" (Bowers and Heilman 1980, see Jewell and McCourt 2000 for a review). Consistent with the pseudoneglect phenomenon, also on the landmark task, when judging lines pre-bisected to the left of their true center, normal participants consider the left segment as being longer than the right one (Milner et al. 1992). This asymmetry likely results from the specialization of networks in the right hemisphere for the deployment of spatial attention (Heilman and Van Den Abell 1980; McCourt and Jewell 1999; Mesulam 1999; Thiebaut de Schotten et al. 2011), although reading habits may also contribute by biasing left-to-right readers so that they explore the line from its left endpoint (Chokron and Imbert 1993). The leftward exploration bias could then lead to a (slight) overestimation of the left segment of the line (see below), consistent with the pseudoneglect asymmetry.

This evidence from normal and brain-damaged patients suggests that spatial attention influences the perceptual estimation of horizontal lengths, leading to over-estimation of the portion of the line where attention is focused. For example, Marshall and Halligan (1990) proposed that during line bisection neglect patients search the line for its midpoint from the right to the left and subsequently place the bisection point where the two hemi-segments appear to be of equal length. A right-ward attentional bias might thus increase the perceptual salience of the right portion relative to the left portion of the line (Anderson 1996), with consequent overestima-tion of the right portion of the line (Urbanski and Bartolomeo 2008), as detailed in the following Sect. 5.3.3.

Toba et al. (2011) investigated the attention determinants of perception of hori-zontal lengths by taking advantage of the attentional repulsion effect (ARE), whereby briefly presented visual stimuli appear displaced away from the focus of attention (Suzuki and Cavanagh 1997). For example, with the horizontal lines used by Toba et al. (2011), attention would perceptually "stretch" the portion of the line that is closer to the cue. The occurrence of an ARE in these conditions in normal subjects would obviously support accounts of neglect patients' biased performance on line bisection as resulting, at least in part, from asymmetric orienting of exoge-nous attention. Observers perceived the transector of pre-bisected lines as being shifted contralaterally to a peripheral visual cue, consistent with the ARE phenom-enon (Suzuki and Cavanagh 1997). Cue-induced exogenous attention repelled the perceived location of the bisection marker away from the attentional focus; as a consequence, observers required the mark to be closer to the attentional focus for it to be judged as lying at the midpoint. In the no-cue condition normal observers often perceived the transector as being situated to the right of its true position, con-sistent with a relative overestimation of the left-sided line segment (pseudoneglect phenomenon). On the other hand, patients' magnification of the right side of the line would subjectively elongate this portion and draw the perceived midpoint of the line rightward into the elongated region. Thus, Toba et al.'s (2011) results provide direct evidence that exogenous orienting of attention (see Sect. 1. 1) can manipulate the perception of horizontal lengths.

5.3.3 Bisecting Imagined Lines: The Endpoint Task

The *endpoint task* was devised by Edoardo Bisiach and his co-workers (Bisiach et al. 1994, 1996). After having performed a traditional bisection task, right-brain-damaged patients were presented with a single dot on a paper sheet and told that it was the center of an imaginary line, similar to those they had been bisecting before. Patients had to mark the right and left endpoints of the imaginary line. Results showed that the distance between the left endpoint and the center was greater than the distance between the center and the right endpoint. Thus, patients tended to reproduce their line bisection errors (although the rightward deviation of the midpoint was smaller than in traditional line bisection). Bisiach and co-workers (Bisiach et al. 1996) interpreted their results as suggesting a distortion of spatial representation in left neglect. Spatial coordinates would display a progressive anisometry or relaxation from the right to the left, such that patients should travel further leftward in order to equalize the amount of perceived spatial extent of the right and left (virtual) segments. Alternatively, however, patients' asymmetry of performance, with a right-sided (virtual) segment shorter than its left counterpart, also remains consistent with the previously described hypothesis of a perceptual asymmetry, leading to an overestimation of the right imagined segment in the context of a competition between the right and the left portions of the imagined line (Marshall and Halligan 1990; Anderson 1996; Toba et al. 2011).

A crucial difference between the anisometry hypothesis and the perceptual competition hypothesis lies in the contribution of the right portion of the line to patients' final performance. According to the competition hypothesis, the right portion of the (virtual or physical) line has an obvious importance in shaping patients' performance, which is based on a perceptual comparison between the two subjective portions of the line. According to the anisometry account, on the other hand, the presence or absence of the right portion should not influence the overshoot of the left endpoint, which results from a relaxation of the relative spatial coordinates.

Consistent with this prediction, Ishiai and his co-workers collected evidence suggesting that the right portion of the line is indeed unimportant to patients' performance. In a first study (Ishiai et al. 2000), neglect patients bisected lines by pointing on a touch panel with a pencillike pointer. Lines of different length (100, 150, or 200 mm) were presented in a random order. There were three conditions: (1) traditional bisection; (2) bisection with cueing, in which patients had to bisect the line after having touched its left endpoint, in order to ensure their perception of the entire line length; (3) "representational" bisection, in which the line disappeared just after the patient had correctly touched its left endpoint; soon afterwards, patients had to touch the midpoint of the just vanished line. Seven patients out of eight deviated more on traditional bisection than on left-cued bisection, consistent with the well-known decrease of rightward errors after left cuing (Riddoch and Humphreys 1983). Interestingly, the "representational" condition evoked similar or greater errors than the left-cueing condition, suggesting that after left cueing the presence of the right segment had no effect on bisection performance and that left neglect occurs mainly for the mental representation of the line.

In a further study, Ishiai and co-workers (2004) asked patients to perform a similar "representational" task. Yet, after having touched the left endpoint, patients were then asked, in different trials, to touch either one of the endpoints or the midpoint of the vanished line. Two patients out of three deviated more rightward on representational bisection than on cued bisection, confirming the previous results and the apparent irrelevance of the right segment of the lines to the final performance. However, it must be noted that several different line lengths were used; as a consequence, patients needed the visual information just presented in order to process each particular line after its disappearance. Thus, the only possible way for patients to perform these "representational" tasks was to make a bisection judgment on the physically presented line before it disappeared. After the line vanished, patients presumably placed the midpoint (or the endpoints) where they remembered them to have been on the physical line. If so, the task could hardly be considered as being purely "representational." Its outcome would rather reflect the patients' (biased) perception of the physical line, including, perhaps crucially, its right portion.

These findings raise important questions regarding functional and neural models of normal space cognition and of left neglect and the understanding of the relationships between visual perception and visual mental imagery. First, is patients' performance on line bisection modulated by the presence/absence of right visual stimuli? Second, how do patients process imagined lines in the presence or absence of either endpoint? Is their performance equivalent to that with physically presented lines (Ishiai et al. 2000, 2004) or can they attain more symmetrical levels of performance in the absence of right-sided, attention-capturing physical stimuli?

To address these issues, Urbanski and Bartolomeo (2008) devised a new test of bisection of printed and imagined lines. They asked normal participants and patients with right-hemisphere lesions and left neglect to set the midpoint and the endpoints of 200-mm lines physically printed on a sheet. Participants had to perform the test either starting from the left or from the right extremity of the line. In separate blocks, participants were presented with blank sheets and were instructed to imagine lines similar to those that they had seen previously and to mark the endpoints and the midpoint of the imagined lines, again starting either from the left or from the right extremity of each imagined line.

The perceptual competition hypothesis predicts greater rightward displacements on the perceptual conditions than on the imagery conditions in neglect patients, because right, non-neglected physical stimuli are important to trigger left neglect (Marshall and Halligan 1990; Anderson 1996; Toba et al. 2011). Deviation should be minimized in the imagery condition with left-to-right scanning, because no physical right-sided stimuli (other than the sheet margin and the casual distractors present during standard clinical examination in ambient light) are present when patients are placing the midpoint. On the contrary, accounts based on representational impairments (Ishiai et al. 2000, 2004), such as space anisometry (Bisiach et al. 1996), predict the absence of any modulation of patients' performance by physically present right-sided stimuli. Patients should show similar degrees of processing asymmetry, no matter whether the lines are printed or imagined or whether a right-sided endpoint is present or not. The results obtained by Urbanski and Bartolomeo (2008) showed that patients had either normal performance or a reversed (leftward) bias when setting the endpoints and the center of an imaginary line starting from the left side, consistent with the perceptual competition hypothesis. In particular, the lack of asymmetry of performance in the left-to-right imagery condition runs counter to the spatial anisometry account (Bisiach et al. 1996), because distortions of spatial coordinates should not depend on the presence or absence of a right-sided visual stimulus. Instead, in patients with left homonymous hemianopia, leftward hypermetria occasionally observed in the endpoint task (i.e., patients travelling too far towards the left when marking the left endpoint after having placed the right endpoint and the center) may be understood as a consequence of saccadic overshooting made to move the blind hemifield away and to bring the endpoint position into the seeing hemifield (Doricchi and Angelelli 1999; Doricchi et al. 2003). This process might result in patients "confabulating" a longer left segment (Chatterjee 2002).

5.3.4 Length Reproduction and Estimation

One important question concerning spatial attention in neglect is, are rightward attentional capture and leftward orienting deficits two (consecutive) sides of the same coin, or should they be considered as distinct components of neglect behavior? To answer this question, Charras et al. (2010) asked neglect patients to draw the horizontal segment of left- or right-directed Ls, on the basis of a given vertical segment (Fig. 5.5a).

Neglect patients drew longer left-directed segments than right-directed segments. However, comparison with controls' performance revealed that neglect patients did overextend horizontal lines towards the left, but did not under-extend rightward lines. This result invites the conclusion that the left–right imbalance observed in length estimation resulted more from left impairment in stimulus processing than from right attentional capture. However, as described above, in a different series of patients, Urbanski and Bartolomeo (2008) found that right attentional capture exerted by the right extremity of horizontal lines did have an important role in patients' performance in bisection-related tasks. Their patients were selected on the basis of the presence of a pathological rightward deviation on line bisection. However, when they had to set the left endpoint of an imaginary line on the basis of a central point, their performance depended on the presence/absence of a (presumably attention-capturing) right endpoint. The two virtual segments were asymmetric, mimicking ordinary line bisection, when the right endpoint was visible, but much more symmetrical when it was not. To account for the apparent discrepancy between the outcome of these two studies, Charras et al. (2010) noted that in their L-shaped figures there was no right-sided horizontal line whose extremity could capture patients' attention, which presumably led to the absence of right overestimation.

In a second study, Charras et al. (2012) were able to confirm and refine their previous conclusions. Patients were asked to estimate the length of left- and right-sided segments with L-, T-, or cross-shaped (X) configurations (Fig. 5.5b). When there was no competition between left and right horizontal segments, such as in the L configurations, the left–right imbalance resulted from left underestimation, in the absence of right overestimation, thus confirming the previous results (Charras et al. 2010). Similar results occurred with the T configurations, when emphasis was put on the vertical dimension of the stimulus (as shown by participants' strong tendency to overestimate the vertical portion of the stimulus), thus presumably preventing left–right integration of the horizontal segments. However, when left and right segments competed to be integrated in a single percept, as in the X configurations, then right attentional capture did contribute to patients' performance. Interestingly, the

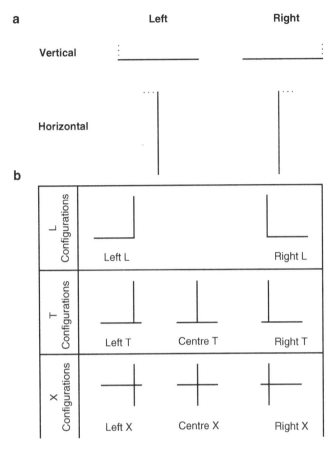

Fig. 5.5 (**a**) Schematic depiction of the stimuli used by Charras et al. (2010). A single *black line*, either horizontal or vertical (40 mm long, 1 mm thick), was printed in the center of the sheet. Participants performed a line extension task in which they were to draw either a horizontal or a vertical line to complete an L figure. The missing line was located either to the left or to the right of the presented line. The position of the missing line was indicated by three small black dots. (**b**) Schematic depiction of the stimuli used by Charras et al. (2012). The L configurations enabled the test of leftward and rightward biases separately. In the T and X configurations, there was a left/right competition between the horizontal line segments left and right of the bisection line. The results showed that in the T configuration the vertical line was overestimated, while in the X configuration the horizontal line was overestimated

presence of left homonymous hemianopia worsened left underestimations, but did not modulate right overestimations.

Based on these results, Charras et al. (2012) proposed the existence of distinct neural bases for right overestimation, resulting from the activity of an isolated left hemisphere (see Sect. 7.4), and left underestimation, dependent on impaired functioning of right-hemisphere attentional networks (Sect. 7.3). In different patients, these two component deficits might have different weights, perhaps depending on individual differences in anatomical asymmetries of frontoparietal networks linked by SLF II and III (Thiebaut de Schotten et al. 2011).

5.4   Variants of Representational Tasks

5.4.1   Problems with Place Descriptions

A basic problem with the description from memory of known places mentioned in Sect. 4.6 is that patients might use abilities other than visual imagery to perform this task. Typically, patients are invited to imagine the places "as if they were in front of them" (Bartolomeo et al. 1994). Despite these instructions, some patients might simply have produced a list of items from verbal semantic memory. If so, imaginal neglect would be underestimated in these tasks and might thus ultimately appear to be less common than visuospatial neglect, whereas the two disorders would in fact have a similar frequency. On the other hand, even when naming an imagined detail, participants could then verbally associate this detail with others nearby, which would thus be mentioned without being imagined (e.g., when describing a map of France, Paris could be verbally associated with the Seine river). If so, there could be a local inflation of details, which would also complicate estimates of frequency of imaginal neglect (Bartolomeo et al. 2005). The issue is of theoretical importance, because if imaginal neglect occurs with an equal or greater frequency than visual neglect, then the two deficits might share a common mechanism, such as the loss of the left part of a putative mental representation of space (Bisiach 1993). On the other hand, a greater frequency of visual than imaginal neglect across patients would be consistent rather with an attentional impairment typically affecting visual objects and in some cases imagined items as well (Bartolomeo et al. 1994). A third possibility is that these two forms of neglect result from entirely different disorders. This possibility is consistent with reports of double dissociations between imaginal and visual neglect (Guariglia et al. 1993; Coslett 1997; Ortigue et al. 2001; Denis et al. 2002), but increases the need for explanation.

Bartolomeo et al. (2005) also listed further problems for place descriptions. Idiosyncratic responses are possible, depending, for example, on the patient's place of residency or vacation. There is a strong influence of premorbid cultural level. Often, too few items are available for statistical analysis. Finally, there is no way to know where patients place the center of their mental images and consequently on which side the produced items are situated in the patient's mental map of space. For example, a lateralized item just imagined could easily become the center of further exploration.

To deal with these issues, other experimental tests of lateralized imaginal abilities have been developed. Denis et al. (2002) presented patients with visual layouts or verbal descriptions of layouts and subsequently asked them to recall the presented material (see also Halligan et al. 1992). Neglect patients reported fewer items from the left than from the right side in both conditions, but especially in the "memory after perception" condition, which resulted in a significant interaction between conditions. However, in the "memory after perception" condition, visual neglect could have biased the perceptual apprehension of the visual scene, consistent with the increased neglect demonstrated in this condition. On the other hand, in the "memory after description" condition, normal controls also had a tendency to report fewer items from the left than from the right side, which might suggest a task-dependent bias.

5.4.2 Mental Line Bisection

Neglect patients may also deviate rightward on the mental bisection of number intervals; for example, when asked which is the median number between 11 and 19, they may answer "17" (Zorzi et al. 2006). In this domain as well, visual and imaginal performance may dissociate. Biased performance with mental number lines might be related to concomitant prefrontal damage and spatial working memory impairment (Doricchi et al. 2005). It would indeed be surprising to find that all neglect patients demonstrate such a mental bias, given that people do not always imagine numbers in spatial arrangements, and even when they do, their mental diagrams are not necessarily oriented along the horizontal direction (Galton 1880).

5.4.3 Imaginal Response Times

Bartolomeo et al. (2005) developed an RT task for imagined locations and compared performance on this task to the widely used task of describing an imaginary map of France (Rode et al. 1995). Participants heard the spoken names of geographical locations (towns and regions of France) and had to press a left- or a right-sided key according to the corresponding imagined location in a mentally generated map of France with Paris as its center. Participants had no obvious way of performing this task without conjuring up a visual mental image of a map of France, because geographical locations are rarely understood in terms of being situated to the "left" or "right" of Paris. Indeed, a subsequent eye movement study (Bourlon et al. 2011a) using the same paradigm in normal participants demonstrated a tendency to produce spontaneous eye movements consistent with the position of the imagined targets, thus suggesting the use of visuospatial processes in this task. By providing participants with the place names, instead of asking them to list the names, the influence of particular cultural backgrounds should be minimized. The imaginal RT task enabled the recording of two measurements, response time and accuracy, that should allow a finer quantitative evaluation of patients' performance than place descriptions. Finally, an imaginary center of the mental map was supplied on each trial by asking participants to start their exploration from the imagined location of Paris.

Twelve control participants and 12 right-brain-damaged patients, of whom 7 had visual neglect, participated in the experiment. Controls and non-neglect patients performed symmetrically. Neglect patients were slower for left than for right imagined locations. On single-case analysis, two patients with visual neglect showed an unequivocal RT asymmetry on the geographical task, but with symmetrical accuracy. The dissociation between response times and accuracy suggests that, in these patients, the left side of the mental map of space was not lost, but only "explored" less efficiently.

However, dissociations between perceptual and imaginal neglect are typically investigated by using very different tasks (e.g., visual target cancellation vs. place descriptions). To address this issue, Bourlon et al. (2008) explored patients' performance on imaginal and perceptual tasks which shared identical stimuli and procedure, except for the modality of stimulus presentation. In different tasks, participants either saw towns/regions on a map of France or heard their names (Bartolomeo et al. 2005) and pressed one of two keys according to the stimulus location (left or right of Paris). A group of 25 neglect patients was less accurate for left-sided stimuli in both modalities; however, the perceptual task elicited a much greater asymmetry of performance on both RTs and response accuracy than the imaginal task did. Moreover, on single-case analysis only one patient with perceptual neglect had asymmetric imaginal accuracy. These findings add to the abundant evidence showing that neglect is more frequent and severe for "real" visual stimuli than for mental images (see Bartolomeo 2002). Thus, also when assessed by using strictly comparable tests, in most cases neglect appears to affect the patients' interaction with the external world, rather than putative mental representations of space (Urbanski and Bartolomeo 2008).

In a further study with the geographical RT task, Bourlon et al. (2011b) asked 19 patients with right brain damage and 12 healthy controls to say whether an auditorily presented French geographical location was left or right of Paris and this time recorded their vocal RTs, instead of manual RTs. Afterwards, participants performed a similar test with visually presented items. Although several patients showed asymmetries of performance on the perceptual version of the test, only one patient was more accurate for right-sided than for left-sided imagined stimuli, thus showing evidence for imaginal neglect. However, this patient performed normally on place description and on mental number line bisection, perhaps as a consequence of different strategies he employed for these tasks. Intriguingly, in this patient sample, the spontaneous description of the map of France gave little evidence for imaginal neglect. Two patients (one with neglect and one without neglect on paper-and-pencil tests) had asymmetric performance consistent with left imaginal neglect, but three others (one with and two without perceptual neglect) had the opposite pattern of performance, with more items described on the left imagined side than on the right side. In contrast, patients' performance on the perceptual RT task was broadly consistent with the outcome of paper-and-pencil tests.

One possibility to account for the rarity of imaginal neglect in this study is that this form of neglect might depend on deficits of top-down processes, such as endogenous attention or active rehearsal of spatial knowledge, which are less impaired than exogenous attention in patients with perceptual neglect (Bartolomeo et al. 1994). If so, the geographical RT task, based on externally provided items, might be too passive a test to frequently elicit imaginal neglect. A novel contribution of the Bourlon et al.'s (2011b) study is that this pattern of results was unlikely to depend on methodological confounds such as lateralized motor response biases (see Sect. 6.3.2) or to result from problems of description from memory, such as the use of nonspatial strategies.

Further evidence on the influence of attentional processes on imaginal neglect was gathered by Loetscher and Brugger (2007), who asked a patient to use a black touch screen to represent the night sky and to touch the locations occupied by (imaginary) stars. The patient placed significantly more stars to the right of the screen midline and then especially when the stars remained illuminated after the touch. If the screen remained black, the asymmetry was less evident. This again suggests an attention-capturing influence of real right-sided visual stimuli on patients' neglect (Bartolomeo et al. 2004; Chokron et al. 2004). But perceptual influences on spatial imagery seem less relevant for casual, task-unrelated stimuli. When patients were asked to imagine and describe the map of France with eyes open or blindfolded, performance was similar regardless of the condition (Rode et al. 2007, 2010) (Fig. 5.6).

5.4.4   REMs in Neglect

Finally, dreaming is a condition which shares with mental imagery a rich visual phenomenology in the absence of any external stimulations. Interestingly, during sleep neglect patients may show suppression of leftward-directed rapid eye movements (REMs) (Doricchi et al. 1991, 1993). Also, a patient with left visual neglect

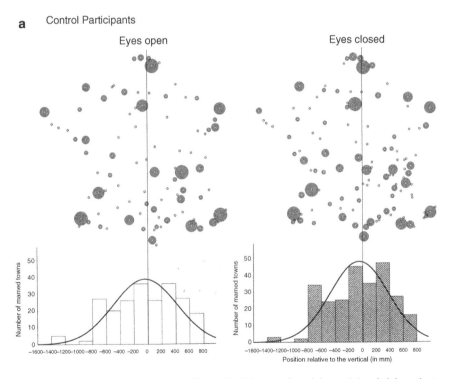

Fig. 5.6 Mental evocation of the map of France in eight control participants (**a**) and eight patients with left neglect (**b**) with eyes open or eyes closed (Rode et al. 2007). Each *circle* indicates the location of a named town on a tracing of the map. For each town, the size of the circle reflects the number of repetitions for all control participants and patients with neglect. *Bottom panels*: distribution of named towns according to their position (in mm) relative to the vertical meridian line. The presence/absence of visual input had no effect on the severity of imaginal neglect in these patients (Reproduced from Rode et al. (2007). © 2007, with permission from Wolters Kluwer Health)

b   Neglect patients

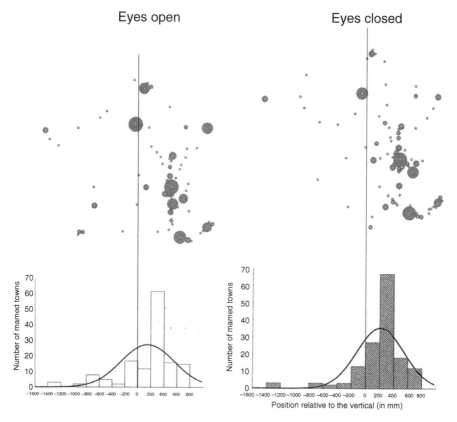

Fig. 5.6 (continued)

and frequent nystagmoid REMs with alternating leftward slow/rightward fast phases, corresponding to dreams with consistent visual events such as a train running leftward, had virtually no nystagmoid REMs in the opposite direction (Doricchi et al. 2006).

5.5   Dissociations in Performance Within and Between Patients

Visual neglect is not a homogeneous condition. Different patients may exhibit distinct patterns of performance (Bartolomeo and Chokron 2001). This has led some authors to propose that neglect as a construct is "a meaningless entity" (Halligan and Marshall 1992). Dissociated pattern of performance in neglect may depend on damage to distinct brain modules (Verdon et al. 2010) or networks (Bartolomeo et al. 2007). For example, patients may neglect left-sided targets on cancellation tasks but accurately bisect horizontal lines or explore the whole cancellation sheet but deviate rightward on line bisection (Binder et al. 1992). However, attentional deficits are often prominent in neglect patients, who characteristically show a bias in spatial orienting favoring ipsilesional (typically right-sided) events over contralesional (left-sided) events, as well as deficits in nonspatial forms of attention such as alerting (see Chap. 6).

As mentioned previously, a possible source of (spurious) dissociations may result from patients learning to use compensatory strategies in one domain but not in another. This occurrence may be difficult or impossible to ascertain; functional dissociations with corresponding lesional differences (e.g., Binder et al. 1992; Doricchi et al. 2005) seem best suited to substantiate claims for different underlying causes. However, it has proven difficult to find a clear correspondence between behavioral dissociations and different lesion localizations, perhaps because clinical, low-definition images are often used, and the focus has mainly been on gray matter lesions, rather than on large-scale brain networks connected by long-range white matter tracts (Bartolomeo et al. 2007; Bartolomeo 2012). Different patterns of disconnection of long-range (Bartolomeo et al. 2007) or short-range (Thiebaut de Schotten et al. 2012) white matter pathways may influence patients' behavior by precluding the access of information to specific brain modules or networks or by preventing the action of compensatory mechanisms based, for example, on left hemisphere systems (see Sect. 6.1.6).

References

Anderson B. Spared awareness for the left side of internal visual images in patients with left-sided extrapersonal neglect. Neurology. 1993;43:213–6.

Anderson B. A mathematical model of line bisection behaviour in neglect. Brain. 1996;119:841–50.

Bartolomeo P. The relationship between visual perception and visual mental imagery: a reappraisal of the neuropsychological evidence. Cortex. 2002;38:357–78.

Bartolomeo P. The elusive nature of white matter damage in anatomo-clinical correlations. Front Hum Neurosci. 2012;6:229.

Bartolomeo P, Chokron S. Levels of impairment in unilateral neglect. In: Boller F, Grafman J, editors. Handbook of neuropsychology. 2nd ed. Amsterdam: Elsevier Science Publishers; 2001. p. 67–98.

Bartolomeo P, D'Erme P, Gainotti G. The relationship between visuospatial and representational neglect. Neurology. 1994;44:1710–4.

Bartolomeo P, Urbanski M, Chokron S, Chainay H, Moroni C, Siéroff E, Belin C, Halligan P. Neglected attention in apparent spatial compression. Neuropsychologia. 2004;42:49–61.

Bartolomeo P, Bachoud-Lévi A-C, Azouvi P, Chokron S. Time to imagine space: a chronometric exploration of representational neglect. Neuropsychologia. 2005;43:1249–57.

Bartolomeo P, Thiebaut de Schotten M, Doricchi F. Left unilateral neglect as a disconnection syndrome. Cereb Cortex. 2007;45:3127–48.

Binder J, Marshall R, Lazar R, Benjamin J, Mohr JP. Distinct syndromes of hemineglect. Arch Neurol. 1992;49:1187–94.

Bisiach E. Mental representation in unilateral neglect and related disorders. Q J Exp Psychol. 1993;46A:435–61.

Bisiach E, Rusconi ML, Peretti VA, Vallar G. Challenging current accounts of unilateral neglect. Neuropsychologia. 1994;32:1431–4.

Bisiach E, Pizzamiglio L, Nico D, Antonucci G. Beyond unilateral neglect. Brain. 1996;119:851–7.

Bourlon C, Pradat-Diehl P, Duret C, Azouvi P, Bartolomeo P. Seeing and imagining the "same" objects in unilateral neglect. Neuropsychologia. 2008;46:2602–6.

Bourlon C, Oliviero B, Wattiez N, Pouget P, Bartolomeo P. Visual mental imagery: what the head's eye tells the mind's eye. Brain Res. 2011a;1367:287–97.

Bourlon C, Duret C, Pradat-Diehl P, Azouvi P, Loeper-Jény C, Merat-Blanchard M, Levy C, Chokron S, Bartolomeo P. Vocal response times to real and imagined stimuli in spatial neglect: a group study and single-case report. Cortex. 2011b;47:536–46.

Bowers D, Heilman KM. Pseudoneglect: effects of hemispace on a tactile line bisection task. Neuropsychologia. 1980;18:491–8.

Charras P, Lupiáñez J, Bartolomeo P. Assessing the weights of visual neglect: a new approach to dissociate defective symptoms from productive phenomena in length estimation. Neuropsychologia. 2010;48:3371–5.

Charras P, Lupiáñez J, Migliaccio R, Toba MN, Pradat-Diehl P, Duret C, Bartolomeo P. Dissecting the component deficits of perceptual imbalance in visual neglect: evidence from horizontal-vertical length comparisons. Cortex. 2012;48:540–52.

Chatterjee A. Spatial anisometry and representational release in neglect. In: Karnath HO, Milner D, Vallar G, editors. The cognitive and neural bases of spatial neglect. Oxford: Oxford University Press; 2002. p. 167–80.

Chokron S, Imbert M. Influence of reading habits on line bisection. Cogn Brain Res. 1993;1:219–22.

Chokron S, Colliot P, Bartolomeo P. The role of vision in spatial representation. Cortex. 2004; 40:281–90.

Coslett HB. Neglect in vision and visual imagery: a double dissociation. Brain. 1997;120:1163–71.

Cristinzio C, Bourlon C, Pradat-Diehl P, Trojano L, Grossi D, Chokron S, Bartolomeo P. Representational neglect in "invisible" drawing from memory. Cortex. 2009;45:313–7.

Denis M, Beschin N, Logie RH, Della Sala S. Visual perception and verbal descriptions as sources for generating mental representations: evidence from representational neglect. Cogn Neuropsychol. 2002;19:97–112.

Doricchi F, Angelelli P. Misrepresentation of horizontal space in left unilateral neglect: role of hemianopia. Neurology. 1999;52:1845–52.

Doricchi F, Guariglia C, Paolucci S, Pizzamiglio L. Disappearance of leftward rapid eye movements during sleep in left visual hemi-inattention. Neuroreport. 1991;2:285–8.

Doricchi F, Guariglia C, Paolucci S, Pizzamiglio L. Disturbances of the rapid eye movements (REMs) of REM sleep in patients with unilateral attentional neglect: clue for the understanding of the functional meaning of REMs. Electroencephalogr Clin Neurophysiol. 1993;87:105–16.

Doricchi F, Guariglia P, Figliozzi F, Magnotti L, Gabriele G. Retinotopic modulation of space misrepresentation in unilateral neglect: evidence from quadrantanopia. J Neurol Neurosurg Psychiatry. 2003;74:116–9.

Doricchi F, Guariglia P, Gasparini M, Tomaiuolo F. Dissociation between physical and mental number line bisection in right hemisphere brain damage. Nat Neurosci. 2005;8:1663–5.

Doricchi F, Iaria G, Silvetti M, Figliozzi F, Siegler I. The "ways" we look at dreams: evidence from unilateral spatial neglect (with an evolutionary account of dream bizarreness). Exp Brain Res. 2006;178:450–61.

Gainotti G, D'Erme P, Bartolomeo P. Early orientation of attention toward the half space ipsilateral to the lesion in patients with unilateral brain damage. J Neurol Neurosurg Psychiatry. 1991;54:1082–9.

Galton F. Visualised numerals. Nature. 1880;21:252–6.

Guariglia C, Padovani A, Pantano P, Pizzamiglio L. Unilateral neglect restricted to visual imagery. Nature. 1993;364:235–7.

Halligan PW, Marshall JC. Left visuospatial neglect: a meaningless entity? Cortex. 1992;28:525–35.

Halligan PW, Marshall JC, Wade DT. Contrapositioning in a case of visual neglect. Neuropsychol Rehabil. 1992;2:125–35.

Harvey M, Milner AD, Roberts RC. An investigation of hemispatial neglect using the landmark task. Brain Cogn. 1995;27:59–78.

Heilman KM, Van Den Abell T. Right hemisphere dominance for attention: the mechanism underlying hemispheric asymmetries of inattention (neglect). Neurology. 1980;30:327–30.

Husain M, Mannan S, Hodgson T, Wojciulik E, Driver J, Kennard C. Impaired spatial working memory across saccades contributes to abnormal search in parietal neglect. Brain. 2001;124: 941–52.

Ishiai S, Koyama Y, Seki K, Izawa M. Line versus representational bisections in unilateral spatial neglect. J Neurol Neurosurg Psychiatry. 2000;69:745–50.

Ishiai S, Koyama Y, Nakano N, Seki K, Nishida Y, Hayashi K. Image of a line is not shrunk but neglected. Absence of crossover in unilateral spatial neglect. Neuropsychologia. 2004;42:251–6.

Jewell G, McCourt ME. Pseudoneglect: a review and meta-analysis of performance factors in line bisection tasks. Neuropsychologia. 2000;38:93–110.

Khurshid S, Trupe LA, Newhart M, Davis C, Molitoris JJ, Medina J, Leigh R, Hillis AE. Reperfusion of specific cortical areas is associated with improvement in distinct forms of hemispatial neglect. Cortex. 2012;48:530–9.

Loetscher T, Brugger P. A disengagement deficit in representational space. Neuropsychologia. 2007;45:1299–304.

Malhotra P, Jager HR, Parton A, Greenwood R, Playford ED, Brown MM, Driver J, Husain M. Spatial working memory capacity in unilateral neglect. Brain. 2005;128:424–35.

Malhotra PA, Soto D, Li K, Russell C. Reward modulates spatial neglect. J Neurol Neurosurg Psychiatry. 2013;84(4):366–9.

Mark VW, Kooistra CA, Heilman KM. Hemispatial neglect affected by non-neglected stimuli. Neurology. 1988;38:1207–11.

Marshall JC, Halligan PW. Line bisection in a case of visual neglect: psychophysical studies with implications of theory. Cogn Neuropsychol. 1990;7:107–30.

McCourt ME, Jewell G. Visuospatial attention in line bisection: stimulus modulation of pseudoneglect. Neuropsychologia. 1999;37:843–55.

Mesulam MM. Attention, confusional states and neglect. In: Mesulam MM, editor. Principles of behavioral neurology. Philadelphia: F.A. Davis; 1985. p. 125–68.

Mesulam M-M. Spatial attention and neglect: parietal, frontal and cingulate contributions to the mental representation and attentional targeting of salient extrapersonal events. Philos Trans R Soc Lond B Biol Sci. 1999;354:1325–46.

Milner AD, Brechmann M, Pagliarini L. To halve and to halve not: an analysis of line bisection judgements in normal subjects. Neuropsychologia. 1992;30:515–26.

Milner AD, Harvey M, Roberts RC, Forster SV. Line bisection errors in visual neglect: misguided action or size distortion? Neuropsychologia. 1993;31:39–49.

Ortigue S, Viaud-Delmon I, Annoni JM, Landis T, Michel C, Blanke O, Vuilleumier P, Mayer E. Pure representational neglect after right thalamic lesion. Ann Neurol. 2001;50:401–4.

Ota H, Fujii T, Suzuki K, Fukatsu R, Yamadori A. Dissociation of body-centered and stimulus-centered representations in unilateral neglect. Neurology. 2001;57:2064–9.

Riddoch MJ, Humphreys GW. The effect of cueing on unilateral neglect. Neuropsychologia. 1983;21:589–99.

Rode G, Perenin MT, Boisson D. Négligence de l'espace représenté : mise en évidence par l'évocation mentale de la carte de France [Neglect of the representational space: demonstration by mental evocation of the map of France]. Rev Neurol. 1995;151:161–4.

Rode G, Revol P, Rossetti Y, Boisson D, Bartolomeo P. Looking while imagining: the influence of visual input on representational neglect. Neurology. 2007;68:432–7.

Rode G, Cotton F, Revol P, Jacquin-Courtois S, Rossetti Y, Bartolomeo P. Representation and disconnection in imaginal neglect. Neuropsychologia. 2010;48:2903–11.

Suzuki S, Cavanagh P. Focused attention distorts visual space: an attentional repulsion effect. J Exp Psychol Hum Percept Perform. 1997;23:443–63.

Thiebaut de Schotten M, Dell'Acqua F, Forkel SJ, Simmons A, Vergani F, Murphy DGM, Catani M. A lateralized brain network for visuospatial attention. Nat Neurosci. 2011;14:1245–6.

Thiebaut de Schotten M, Tomaiuolo F, Aiello M, Merola S, Silvetti M, Lecce F, Bartolomeo P, Doricchi F. Damage to white matter pathways in sub-acute and chronic spatial neglect: a group study and two single-case studies with complete virtual "in-vivo" tractography dissection. Cereb Cortex. 2012 (Still in press).

Toba MN, Cavanagh P, Bartolomeo P. Attention biases the perceived midpoint of horizontal lines. Neuropsychologia. 2011;49:238–346.

Urbanski M, Bartolomeo P. Line bisection in left neglect: the importance of starting right. Cortex. 2008;44:782–93.

Verdon V, Schwartz S, Lovblad KO, Hauert CA, Vuilleumier P. Neuroanatomy of hemispatial neglect and its functional components: a study using voxel-based lesion-symptom mapping. Brain. 2010;133:880–94.

Wojciulik E, Rorden C, Clarke K, Husain M, Driver J. Group study of an "undercover" test for visuospatial neglect: invisible cancellation can reveal more neglect than standard cancellation. J Neurol Neurosurg Psychiatry. 2004;75:1356–8.

Zorzi M, Priftis K, Meneghello F, Marenzi R, Umiltà C. The spatial representation of numerical and non-numerical sequences: evidence from neglect. Neuropsychologia. 2006;44:1061–7.

Further Reading

Aiello M, Jacquin-Courtois S, Merola S, Ottaviani T, Tomaiuolo F, Bueti D, Rossetti Y, Doricchi F. No inherent left and right side in human 'mental number line': evidence from right brain damage. Brain. 2013;135(Pt 8):2492–505.

Binder J, Marshall R, Lazar R, Benjamin J, Mohr JP. Distinct syndromes of hemineglect. Arch Neurol. 1992;49(11):1187–94.

Marshall J, Halligan PW. Whoever would have imagined it? Bisiach and Luzzatti (1978) on representational neglect in patients IG and NV. In: Code C, Wallesch CW, Joanette Y, Roch Lecours A, editors. Classic cases in neuropsychology II, vol. 2. Hove: Taylor & Francis Books Ltd; 2002. p. 272–4.

Milner AD, Harvey M. Distortion of size perception in visuospatial neglect. Curr Biol. 1995;5(1):85–9.

Chapter 6
Component Deficits of Neglect

Keywords Attentional capture • Disengagement deficit • Response bias • Directional hypokinesia • Spatial working memory • Nonlateralized deficits

The possible mechanisms leading to neglect behavior have fostered a considerable debate. The general lack of consensus may depend on several factors, including inadequate theoretical understanding of visuospatial functions, important interindividual differences among patients, and the possibility that several independent deficits, probably interacting with each other, may contribute to neglect signs. In the last decades, research on neglect is shifting from the description of dissociations in patients' performance to the dissection of putative component deficits of neglect and of their modes of interaction. Not all of these putative component deficits need be present in all patients; distinct combination of deficits may give rise to peculiar patterns of neglect behavior in different patients (Coulthard et al. 2007). Possible component deficits in neglect include impaired orienting of spatial attention (Bartolomeo and Chokron 2002), defective building or maintenance of spatial representations (Bisiach 1993), and difficulties in programming left-directed hand movements (Coulthard et al. 2007).

It is also possible, however, that not all these putative deficits have similar weights in all patients. Clinically, some deficits may be more frequent or severe than others in shaping patients' behavior. For example, deficits of spatial attention, such as an early engagement of attention towards right-sided, non-neglected items as soon as the visual scene unfolds (Gainotti et al. 1991; D'Erme et al. 1992; Natale et al. 2007; Siéroff et al. 2007), followed by impaired disengagement from these same items (Posner et al. 1984), have often been considered key component deficits of neglect. Importantly, these deficits seem mainly to concern exogenous, or stimulus-related, orienting of attention (see Sect. 1.1), with relative sparing of endogenous, or voluntary, orienting (Bartolomeo et al. 2001a). Thus, the simple presence of right-sided distractors can disrupt patients' performance by capturing their attention (Bartolomeo et al. 2004). Also nonlateralized deficits can contribute, perhaps crucially (Robertson 2001; Husain and Rorden 2003), to clinical neglect.

P. Bartolomeo, *Attention Disorders After Right Brain Damage*,
DOI 10.1007/978-1-4471-5649-9_6, © Springer-Verlag London 2014

For example, patients with left neglect can be impaired in processing not only left-sided objects but also items presented in central (Husain et al. 1997; Malhotra et al. 2005) or right-sided locations (Bartolomeo and Chokron 1999; Bartolomeo et al. 1999; Rusconi et al. 2002; Snow and Mattingley 2006; Bourgeois et al. 2012). However, attention deficits may occur after right brain damage even in the absence of clinical neglect (Posner et al. 1984; Bartolomeo 1997; Habekost and Rostrup 2007). This evidence is consistent with the above-stated hypothesis that several deficits concur to produce overt neglect behavior (Gainotti et al. 1991; Bartolomeo 2007; Coulthard et al. 2007).

6.1 Spatial Attention

As described in Chap. 1, spatial orienting requires the integrated activity of brain networks with prefrontal and parietal cortical nodes and with important hemispheric differences favoring the right hemisphere. The work of Michael Posner and co-workers (see Posner 1980, for review) has made a major contribution to our understanding of the functioning of spatial attention. The cued detection task developed by Posner and co-workers (see Sect. 1.1) has had a major impact in the literature on normal attention and its deficits.

6.1.1 Early Ipsilesional Capture and the Disengagement Deficit

Posner, Walker, Friedrich, and Rafal (1984) asked six right-brain-damaged and seven left-brain-damaged patients with predominantly parietal lesions to perform their cued detection task. Cues were either central or peripheral, but always informative of the future target location; 80 % of cues were valid and 20 % invalid. Patients were disproportionally slow when a target occurring on the side opposite to the brain lesion was preceded by an invalid ipsilesional cue. This RT pattern was present in patients with right and left hemisphere lesions, but considerably larger in right-brain-damaged patients and evident with both central and peripheral cues. Posner et al. (1984) termed this effect "extinction-like RT pattern" because it was reminiscent of extinction of contralesional stimuli in double visual stimulation (see Sect. 2.2) and argued that it resulted from an impaired disengagement of attention from the ipsilesional side, when attention had to move to a contralesional target (Posner et al. 1987). This notion may be used to explain the behavior of patients suffering from unilateral neglect; these patients would neglect the contralesional side of space because their attention cannot easily disengage from ipsilesional objects. However, the parietal patients in the Posner et al. (1984) study showed little or no neglect on paper-and-pencil tests (no neglect in five patients, minimal neglect in two, mild in five, and moderate in one). Thus, in this study there was no direct evidence for a relationship between the observed extinction-like RT pattern and neglect.

Morrow and Ratcliff (1988) tested 12 patients with right hemisphere lesions and ten left-brain-damaged patients using an RT paradigm with peripheral informative cues (75 % of the cues were valid and 25 % invalid). All patients had lesions including the parietal lobe, contralesional neglect, or both. Only right-brain-damaged patients showed a significant extinction-like RT pattern. The observed cost for contralesional targets preceded by invalid cues correlated with a measure of left neglect, thus suggesting a causal relationship between the two phenomena.

However, for such a disengage deficit to produce clinical left neglect, attention must logically have been engaged to the right *before* the occurrence of the disengagement problem. D'Erme et al. (1992) found evidence for such an early rightward engagement by manipulating the Posner RT paradigm. They contrasted the traditional task in which targets appeared in boxes (see Fig. 1.1) with a condition in which targets appeared in a blank screen, not surrounded by boxes. The presence of the boxes considerably increased the left/right RT difference for neglect patients, as if the right-sided box acted as an invalid cue for left targets. Thus, the mere appearance on the computer screen of the placeholder boxes elicited a shift of patients' attention towards the rightmost box. Because the boxes were not informative about the future location of the targets, the type of orienting elicited by the boxes could best be characterized as reflexive, or exogenous, as opposed to the voluntary, or endogenous orienting elicited by central cues or by peripheral informative cues (Müller and Rabbitt 1989). Thus, D'Erme et al. (1992) proposed that the attentional imbalance in neglect was primarily one of exogenous attention, in keeping with previous similar suggestions based on the apparent "automaticity" of rightward attentional attraction in left neglect (Gainotti et al. 1991).

Moreover, Posner et al. (1984) used informative cues, thus making it difficult to discriminate between exogenous and endogenous orienting of attention in neglect (see Sect. 1.1.1). Làdavas et al. (1994a) contrasted the effects on target detection of central informative cues (an arrow presented near fixation) with that of peripheral non-informative cues (an arrow presented above one of the placeholder boxes). Results showed that central cues pointing towards the left were able to decrease the number of omissions of left targets in neglect patients, whereas peripheral cues presented on the left side had no significant effect on patients' accuracy. The authors concluded that neglect patients were not able to orient their attention leftward exogenously, but they could do so voluntarily (see also Smania et al. 1998). However, besides their different effects on exogenous and endogenous orienting, central and peripheral cues might act on distinct stages of information processing (an early perceptual stage for peripheral cues, and a late perceptual or a decision stage for central cues: Riggio and Kirsner 1997), thus rendering difficulty in any direct comparison between their respective effects on performance. Moreover, in the case of patients suffering from a spatial bias, the different spatial localization of central and peripheral cues may complicate the interpretation of the results.

Bartolomeo et al. (2001a) explored attentional orienting in left unilateral neglect by using exclusively peripheral cues, whose informative value was systematically

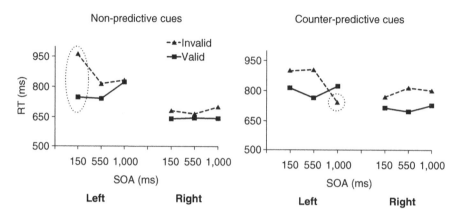

Fig. 6.1 Response times to left- and right-sided targets preceded by invalid or valid peripheral cues with different degrees of predictiveness (Bartolomeo et al. 2001a). In these six neglect patients, the disengagement deficit elicited by 50 % valid cues (*left panel*, dotted ellipse) reverted to an RT advantage with 20 % valid cues (*right panel*, dotted circle)

manipulated. They studied six patients with right hemisphere lesions and signs of left visual neglect on paper-and-pencil tests, as well as age-matched controls. In Experiment 1, cues were non-predictive (50 % valid), and targets could appear either in the cued or in the uncued box with equal probabilities. This situation should evoke a purely exogenous shift of attention towards the cued box (Müller and Rabbitt 1989), particularly at short SOAs (Müller and Findlay 1988). Controls showed slowed RTs to the cued locations at longer SOAs (>150 ms), consistent with the phenomenon of IOR (see Sect. 1.1 above and the next section). Neglect patients had no evidence of IOR for right targets; they showed the typical disengagement deficit discovered by Posner et al. (1984), i.e., a disproportionate cost for left targets preceded by right (invalid) cues; this cost was maximal at the shortest SOA. This feature, together with the non-predictive nature of the cues in this experiment, strongly suggests a biased exogenous orienting in these neglect patients (Fig. 6.1, left panel).

In Experiment 2, 80 % of the cues were valid, i.e., they correctly predicted the location of the impending target, thus inducing an initially exogenous, and later endogenous, attentional shift towards the cued box. Neglect patients showed again a cost for left invalidly cued targets, which this time persisted at SOAs >150 ms, as if patients' attention had been cued to the right side not only exogenously but also endogenously, thus rendering more difficulty in an endogenous reorienting towards the left. In Experiment 3, most cues (80 %) were invalid. In this situation, cues should normally prompt an initial exogenous orienting towards the cued box, later followed by an inhibition of this exogenous shift, to be replaced by an endogenous shift towards the uncued box (Posner et al. 1982). Thus, for long enough SOAs this condition explores endogenous orienting in relative isolation. Controls were able to take advantage of invalid cues to rapidly respond to targets. In this condition, neglect patients were strikingly able to nullify their spatial bias and to reverse the disengage deficit; they achieved their fastest RTs for left targets, which were in the range of their RTs for right targets (see the right panel in Fig. 6.1). However, for neglect patients, fast responses to left targets occurred only at 1,000-ms SOA, while controls were able to redirect their attention to the uncued box already at 550-ms SOA. Thus, the preserved endogenous orienting showed by this group of neglect patients was relatively spared, if slowed.

6.1.2   Ineffective Exploration and Implicit Knowledge

Disturbances of orienting of spatial attention thus seem consistent with several neglect phenomena, provided that these accounts are articulated as an association of a number of concurrent deficits (Bartolomeo and Chokron 2001). However, on some occasions neglect patients do seem to orient towards neglected stimuli, yet fail nevertheless to produce the correct response. For example, Bisiach et al. (1994) observed neglect patients who occasionally followed with their index finger the complete contour of a drawing, but failed to notice the details on its left side. As previously mentioned (see Sect. 4.5.3), when bisecting lines, some patients seem to explore the left part of the line, but this leftward search does not influence the final bisection decision, which remains rightward biased (Ishiai et al. 1996; Barton et al. 1998). Similarly, neglect patients may sometimes fail to produce the appropriate manual response to left-sided stimuli despite having looked at them (Làdavas et al. 1997).

Also difficult to reconcile with purely attentional accounts of neglect are the patterns of performance of those patients who show signs of implicit (or "covert") knowledge of otherwise neglected details, without overt verbal recognition and sometimes with confabulated responses. In these cases, a certain amount of information seems to have been processed by the patient, but perhaps to an insufficient level to grant explicit reportability. Thus, patients with extinction can perform better than chance when forced to make same/different judgments or select in a multiple choice the identity of a non-explicitly detected item (Volpe et al. 1979). Neglect patients can show implicit semantic processing of the stimulus presented in the neglected hemifield (McGlinchey-Berroth et al. 1993; Berti et al. 1994), although perhaps in only a minority of cases (D'Erme et al. 1993). In an impressive case report, Marshall and Halligan (1988) described a patient with severe left neglect and hemianopia who was unable to tell the difference between drawings of two similar, vertically arranged houses, one of which depicted its left side on fire (Fig. 6.2).

However, when asked in which of the two houses she would live, the patient consistently chose the house that was not burning. Another patient (Manning and Kartsounis 1993) chose the non-burning house confabulating that it had an extra fireplace. Similar confabulations were described in a group of 13 neglect patients (Doricchi et al. 1997), who sometimes described the chosen house as being "better" or "bigger."

These patterns of performance are reminiscent of those shown by split-brain patients. In these patients, the left hemisphere, which has no access to information reaching the right hemisphere, sometimes provides post hoc confabulatory verbal explanations of actions performed by the right hemisphere (Gazzaniga and

Fig. 6.2 The burning house experiment. The patient described by Marshall and Halligan (1988) had left neglect and hemianopia. She explicitly denied any differences between the two houses; however, when asked where she would prefer to live, she consistently chose the non-burning house

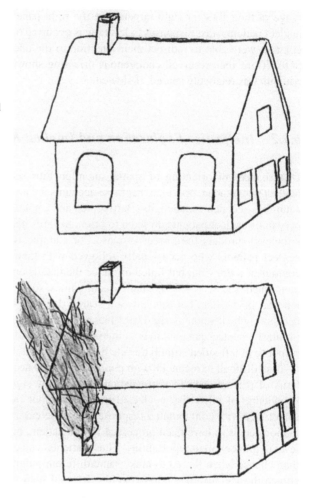

Baynes 2000). It is thus possible that implicit knowledge phenomena in patients with right hemisphere damage depend on interhemispheric disconnection (Bartolomeo et al. 2007), with left-sided information being processed by an isolated right hemisphere, and occasional post hoc confabulations generated by an ill-informed left hemisphere (see Geschwind 1965).

6.1.3 Neglect of Spatial Locations or of Objects in Space?

The disengagement deficit described by Posner and co-workers (1984, 1987) appears to be a stable marker of neglect. Indeed, even if the disengagement deficit is greater in neglect patients with right hemisphere damage, it is also present in patients with left brain damage, but only if they show signs of right neglect (Losier and Klein 2001). Therefore, a causal relationship between the magnitude of the disengagement deficit and the severity of neglect has been suggested (Morrow and Ratcliff 1988; but see Siéroff et al. 2007), despite the fact that disengagement deficit can also be observed in patients without clinical signs of neglect (Posner et al. 1984). Thus, the disengagement deficit can be a valuable marker for clinical assessment of neglect patients, for example, in evaluating the therapeutic effect of rehabilitation strategies (Striemer and Danckert 2007).

The disengagement deficit was originally conceived as a difficulty in disengaging attention "from a location other than the target" (Posner et al. 1984, p. 1872), when attention had to be moved towards the contralesional (left) space (Posner et al. 1987). However, attention can be directed not only to a region of space but also (and perhaps more importantly) to visual objects in space (Egly et al. 1994; Valdes-Sosa et al. 1998). In fact, paying attention to "blank" spatial locations, devoid of any object, can be difficult or impossible for normal participants (see Nakayama and Mackeben 1989, p. 1648). On the other hand, the early attentional capture typical of patients with severe neglect does require a physical object to be presented on the right side (Gainotti et al. 1991; D'Erme et al. 1992). These considerations raise important issues concerning of the nature of the disengagement deficit. Does this deficit reflect a directional deficit of disengaging attention from an ipsilesional to a contralesional location (Posner et al. 1987), or could it better be conceived as an impaired disengagement from visual *objects* presented on the ipsilesional side?

To address this issue, Rastelli et al. (2008) asked normal controls and ten neglect patients to perform a speeded detection task in which targets were preceded by non-informative peripheral cues, but manipulated the nature of the attention-capturing cue. In one condition, the cue consisted of the brightening of one of two lateral boxes (onset cues), whereas in the other condition the cue consisted of the disappearance of one box (offset cues). It has been shown that both types of cues can attract spatial attention and produce standard facilitation effects at short SOAs (Pratt and McAuliffe 2001). Therefore, if neglect patients' disengagement deficit were exclusively spatially based, it should occur even with offset cues. If, on the contrary, the disengagement deficit concerned not space per se, but objects in space, then the disengagement deficit should occur only in, or be increased by, the onset condition. The results obtained by Rastelli et al. (2008) clearly supported this last prediction. A typical disengagement deficit was obtained with onset cues at short SOA, but the disengagement deficit completely disappeared with offset cues (Fig. 6.3).

Except for the overall slowed RTs, neglect patients demonstrated a similar pattern of results as controls in the offset condition at short SOA. Thus, in the absence of a visual stimulus capable of holding their attention on the non-neglected side, neglect patients were able to redirect attention to the neglected side relatively quickly. This result again attests to the special nature of the attention deficit in neglect, which seems not simply related to spatial positions per se, but to the objects that appear in these spatial locations. The privileged status of stimulus onsets, as compared to stimulus offsets, to capture and maintain attention is also consistent

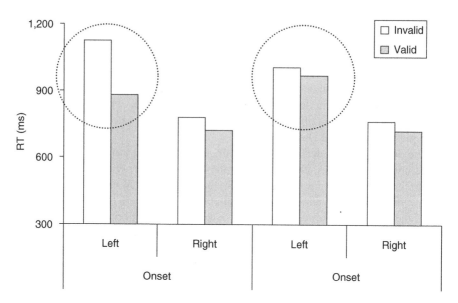

Fig. 6.3 Response times obtained by ten neglect patients for left- and right-sided targets preceded by onset or offset peripheral cues, either invalid or valid, at short (100-ms) SOA (Rastelli et al. 2008). The *dotted circles* highlight the disengagement deficit, which was typical for left invalidly cued targets with onset cues, but virtually disappeared with offset cues

with evidence from visual search tasks in normal participants (see, e.g. Yantis and Jonides 1990).

Thus, Rastelli et al. (2008) demonstrated an important characteristic of the disengagement deficit in neglect patients: the presence of a visual object in which the target appears is a necessary condition for the deficit to emerge. As a consequence, the deficit cannot simply be considered as a directional spatial deficit (Posner et al. 1987). It is right-sided objects (and not spatial regions) that tend to capture patients' attention, consistent with the particular relationships between object-based and exogenous forms of attention (Macquistan 1997). Thus, models of orienting of attention in neglect must take into account the relationship of the disengagement deficit to visual objects in space.

6.1.4 Object-Based Neglect

If spatial attention can be better conceived as orienting towards objects in space than towards "blank" regions of space, then, it should also be possible to observe instances of neglect of the left part of objects, independent of the absolute location of these objects in space. The "piecemeal" copy of complex drawings shown in Fig. 4.9d is an example of such object-based neglect (see Gainotti et al. 1972). It is, however, uncertain whether and to what extent object-based neglect has an independent status (Driver and Pouget 2000). Patients may show such object-based neglect as a sequel of scene-based neglect, when they are starting to recover some capacity of leftward exploration, but the right part of each object continues to capture their attention (Mattingley et al. 1994; Seki et al. 1996; Gainotti et al. 2008). However, evidence from the cancellation test developed by Ota et al. (2001; see Sect. 5.2.3 above) demonstrated dissociations between scene-based and object-based neglect in different patients, with possible anatomical differences (see Sect. 7.5 below).

Another variety of object-based neglect may occur with tilted or rotated stimuli, so that their canonical left part is no longer on the left of the patient's sagittal midline. Thus, patients can be impaired in processing details situated on the left of an object's canonical axis, even when the objects are tilted by 45° towards the right, so that these details are now in the patient's right hemispace (Driver and Halligan 1991; Driver et al. 1994).

Also, a left-handed patient with left hemisphere damage and right neglect produced errors on the final part of words, irrespective of whether the words were presented in a horizontal, vertical, or mirror-reversed format (Caramazza and Hillis 1990). A right-brain-damaged patient, who was also left handed and had a presumably atypical hemispheric asymmetry, developed aphasia and neglect dyslexia for the initial part of words in both horizontal and vertical presentations (Miceli and Capasso 2001). In contrast with these reports, Farah et al. (1990) found no evidence of object-based neglect in a group of ten left neglect patients. When identifying single letters scattered over drawings of familiar objects, patients failed to report left-sided letters when the objects were upright, but they correctly reported these same letters when the objects were tilted. Behrmann and Moscovitch (1994) proposed that object-based neglect might emerge only for those objects which have an intrinsic handedness, where a vertical reference axis allows the definition of left and right with respect to the object itself (see Driver and Halligan 1991). Consistent with this prediction, they demonstrated object-based neglect with uppercase letters presenting a left–right asymmetry (e.g., B, E), but not with symmetrical letters (A, X). Behrmann and Tipper (1999) asked left neglect patients to respond to targets appearing inside one of two horizontally aligned circles of different colors. As expected, patients responded faster to right-sided than to left-sided targets, consistent with scene-based neglect. However, when the two circles were connected by a line, thus forming a single perceptual object like a barbell, and the barbell rotated by 180° just before the target appeared, the effect was reversed. In this case, RTs for the targets now on the left side, but appearing in a previously right-sided circle, were faster than RTs for the targets appearing on the right, thus suggesting object-based neglect. In other words, the *same* neglect patients could show either space- or object-based neglect depending on the experimental conditions. Thus, it is unclear whether all instances of object-based neglect result from distinct deficits or if at least in some cases object-based neglect depends on the strategy adopted by the patient, which would translate a typical egocentric neglect into allocentric neglect based on intrinsic object coordinates.

6.1.5   Neglect and Inhibition of Return

The phenomenon of inhibition of return (IOR, see Sect. 1.1) corresponds to longer response times when processing information from an already inspected spatial
location. IOR occurs both with manual responses (such as a spacebar keypress)
and with saccades to peripheral visual stimuli. Activity in the retinotectal visual
pathway is traditionally considered as being important for IOR (Sapir et al. 1999;
Dorris et al. 2002). Focal lesions (Sapir et al. 1999) or degeneration (Rafal et al.
1988) of the superior colliculi can lead to impaired manual IOR. However, cortical mechanisms also appear to be implicated in IOR. In particular, frontoparietal
networks involved in spatial attention (see Sect. 1.1 above) are plausible candidates
for the cortical control of IOR. For example, experiments with transcranial magnetic stimulation (TMS), which can reversibly and noninvasively "interfere" with
specific cortical regions to probe their implication in the processing underlying a
given ability, found disturbed manual IOR upon stimulation of frontal eye fields
(Ro et al. 2003), IPS (Chica et al. 2011a) and TPJ (Chica et al. 2011a) in the right
hemisphere.

As mentioned before, in neglect patients attention tends to be repeatedly captured by the same right-sided items (Gainotti et al. 1991; Mannan et al. 2005) and
to remain engaged with these stimuli (Posner et al. 1984; Rastelli et al. 2008), with
little or no exploration of the rest of the visual scene. Not surprisingly, then, IOR
can be abnormal in visual neglect (Bartolomeo et al. 1999). When pressing a key in
response to peripheral visual targets which were occasionally repeated on the same
side of space, patients with left neglect presented abnormal facilitation, instead of
IOR, for repeated right-sided items, i.e., for items appearing in their supposedly
normal hemispace (Bartolomeo et al. 1999). Other patients with right hemisphere
damage but without neglect had, instead, normal IOR for both sides of space
(Bartolomeo et al. 1999). These results were later confirmed in neglect patients with
cue–target paradigms (Bartolomeo et al. 2001a; Lupiáñez et al. 2004; Siéroff et al.
2007). Patients with parietal damage also demonstrated decreased IOR (but not
facilitation) on the ipsilesional side, even in the absence of neglect signs (Vivas
et al. 2003, 2006). These results are important in suggesting that cortical networks
including the right parietal lobe (Sect. 1.1.2), which are typically dysfunctional in
neglect patients (Chap. 7), are implicated in the occurrence of IOR. However, in
these studies eye movements were not controlled; if patients looked at ipsilesional
first targets or cues (a frequent occurrence in right-brain-damaged patients, Gainotti
et al. 1991), they received the second stimulus on the fovea. Then fast responses to
foveal stimuli could have offset IOR. Moreover, the level of detail of the anatomical
analysis of lesions in these studies was insufficient to draw firm conclusions about
the identity of the cortical circuits implicated in the modulation of IOR.

To address these issues, Bourgeois et al. (2012) explored both IOR with central fixation and manual responses and IOR generated by saccadic responses in
neglect patients, while eye movements were monitored at all times, by using
a target–target paradigm similar to the one used in the seminal study on IOR in

neglect (Bartolomeo et al. 1999). The manual RT results nicely replicated previous studies (Bartolomeo et al. 1999, 2001a), demonstrating abnormal facilitation, instead of IOR, under covert orienting for right-sided targets in neglect patients. This abnormal facilitation was not restricted to the stimulated location, but spread to the whole right hemispace. Trials in which eye movements had occurred were eliminated from analysis; hence, the observed "facilitation of return" could not depend on eye movement artifacts.

To explain these findings, one might evoke a putative deficit in mechanisms that prioritize spatial representations, inducing a failure to remember which locations have already been examined during visual search (Pisella and Mattingley 2004; Mannan et al. 2005). Such impairment might contribute to neglect signs such as lack of awareness of left-sided events and revisiting behavior (see Sect. 6.4 below). An alternative hypothesis is that the tendency for patients' attention to be automatically and, as it were, "magnetically" captured by right-sided events (see Sect. 6.1.1 above) determines fast processing of events on the right side even when they are presented consecutively (Bartolomeo et al. 1999). If so, then right-sided events might present a perpetual character of "novelty" for neglect patients, thus cancelling IOR.

However, Bourgeois et al. (2012) obtained different results when attention was overtly oriented by asking patients to make saccades towards the targets. In these conditions, neglect patients displayed normal IOR for repeated right-sided targets. For saccadic IOR, there was a central cue back between targets. It is possible that the central cue back was more effective in bringing patients' attention back to the center because attention typically follows eye movements (Shepherd et al. 1986). As a consequence, patients' attention was less likely to be maintained on the right-sided placeholder when the second target occurred, with consequent slower RTs (i.e., IOR) for repeated right-sided targets.

Abnormal IOR observed in neglect patients for right-sided events in covert orienting situations (where manual responses are required) can be explained by a disruption of frontoparietal attention networks with consequent spatial attention deficits (see Chaps. 1 and 7). Consistent with this hypothesis, all the neglect patients in the study by Bourgeois et al. (2012) had damage to the right parietal cortex or to its connections to the ipsilateral prefrontal cortex. Conversely, relatively spared circuits implicating the superior colliculus in the same patients might account for their preserved saccadic IOR because saccadic IOR is more related to the integrity of the retinotectal pathway (Rafal et al. 1989; Dorris et al. 2002). Interestingly, subsequent research (Bourgeois et al. 2013b) on normal participants who received off-line repetitive TMS on the right IPS and the right TPJ found evidence consistent with the patient study, because repetitive TMS interference over both sites lastingly interfered with manual but not saccadic IOR for right-sided targets. Further TMS evidence (Bourgeois et al. 2013a) indicated that comparable stimulation over the IPS or TPJ in the left hemisphere did not produce measurable changes in either manual or saccadic IOR. Thus, similar hemispheric differences seem to exist for cortical control of exogenous attention (Sect. 1.1.2), cortical modulation of IOR, and the occurrence of visuospatial neglect after brain damage.

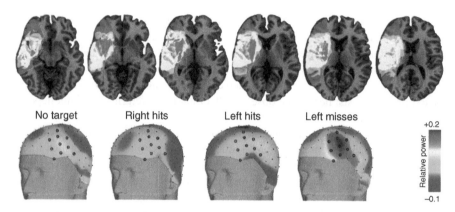

Fig. 6.4 *Top*: lesion overlap for the five patients studied by Rastelli et al. (2013). *Bottom*: the pattern of left prefrontal beta activity which selectively preceded episodes of neglect for left-sided targets (Reproduced from Rastelli et al. (2013). © 2013, with permission from Elsevier)

6.1.6 Neglect and Spontaneous Brain Activity

Neglect patients' performance can be variable and fluctuating over time (Anderson et al. 2000; Bartolomeo et al. 2001b). At chronic post-injury stages, patients may from time to time gain awareness of sufficiently salient visual stimuli, which could be intermittently omitted thereafter (Wade et al. 1988; Small and Ellis 1994). In a similar way, during stimulation near the perceptual threshold, healthy individuals often fail to see stimuli that at other times are readily detectable (Chica et al. 2011b). In these cases, stimulus salience remains constant; thus, such behavioral variability might correlate with the functional state of specific brain regions prior to stimulus onset (Fox and Raichle 2007). In support of this hypothesis, extensive evidence indicate the existence of specific pre-stimulus patterns of activated and deactivated regions, the processing of subsequent stimuli. For instance, pre-stimulus fluctuations of electrophysiological measures (Chica et al. 2010) and hemodynamic signals (Ress et al. 2000; Boly et al. 2007) can predict the subject's ability to acknowledge or not the presence of a subsequently presented stimulus.

Rastelli et al. (2013) took advantage of the high temporal resolution of magneto-encephalography (MEG) recordings to compare the temporal dynamics and brain regional synchrony events before target omissions to the brain events when the very same targets were detected. A group of five right-brain-damaged patients with left neglect performed a go/no-go lateralized detection task. Neural oscillatory activity was explored in the half second preceding target presentation. Results showed a robust pre-stimulus low-beta synchronization (13–17 Hz) over prefrontal sensors in the left, unimpaired hemisphere. The observed pre-stimulus activity only occurred when the (future) response to left-sided targets was eventually omitted (Fig. 6.4).

Thus, in this group of neglect patients, target misses had a neural signature of their own, perhaps corresponding to active processes in the left hemisphere hindering awareness. The observed activity preceded target onset during a time period crucial for attentional orienting (see Sect. 1.1.1 above) and other brain preparatory states and was localized in a remote and anatomically unaffected prefrontal region, in the contralesional hemisphere. Independent support of the hypothesis that left frontal activity may have a bearing on left visuospatial neglect comes from the case report of a patient with typical parietal damage in the right hemisphere, who abruptly recovered from neglect after a subsequent lesion in the left lateral frontal cortex (Vuilleumier et al. 1996). In another study on right-brain-damaged patients (Oliveri et al. 1999), single-pulse TMS interfering with the activity of the left frontal cortex decreased the number of left tactile extinctions induced by the simultaneous electrical stimulation of the right and left fingers. More generally, the finding that left omissions were preceded by a specific pattern of activity in the ipsilateral, non-lesioned hemisphere, supports network-based models of neglect (see Sect. 7.3 below), which postulate that neglect does not directly result from focal brain damage, but depends on dysfunction of large-scale brain networks within and across the two hemispheres. Thus, in brain-damaged patients, target misses may not only be related to lack of the appropriate brain events (Vuilleumier et al. 2001) but may possess a neural signature of their own. In particular, left prefrontal activity patterns could be a correlate of inappropriate rightward orienting of spatial attention during the pre-stimulus period, resulting in inadequate preparation of the brain to respond to left-sided targets. As described in Sect. 1.1, spatial orienting requires the integrated activity of brain networks with prefrontal and parietal cortical nodes, a coordination that could also partly rely on beta-band oscillatory synchrony (Gross et al. 2004; Buschman and Miller 2007).

6.1.7   The Paradox of the Left Hemisphere

One of the many paradoxes of neglect after right hemisphere damage concerns the role of attention networks in the left hemisphere. Left neglect has been shown to decrease with either acute vascular lesion of the healthy left hemisphere (Vuilleumier et al. 1996) or TMS interference on the left parietal lobe (Sect. 9.3 below). This is consistent with evidence correlating neglect with a hyperactivity of these networks relative to their right hemisphere homologues (Corbetta et al. 2005; Koch et al. 2008). However, in other cases neglect recovery seems to correlate with an increase in functioning of left hemisphere attentional networks (Pantano et al. 1992; Perani et al. 1993). Thus, left hemisphere attentional network activity seems to be maladaptive in some cases, but adaptive in others.

To explain these discrepancies, we need more articulated models of intra- and interhemispheric functioning of attentional networks in neglect. A classic model of neglect, the opponent processor model (Kinsbourne 1993), stipulates that left neglect results from a hyperactive left hemisphere, liberated from the inhibitory control exerted by the right hemisphere through callosal connections. Although this may be a plausible model for functioning of subcortical structures such as the superior colliculi (Sprague 1966; Rushmore et al. 2006), understanding callosal interhemispheric interactions as being exclusively inhibitory is clearly an oversimplification (see, e.g. Doty 2003). Callosal connections are likely to exert both excitatory and inhibitory effects (mostly through interneurons) on the opposite hemisphere, much as intra-hemispheric long-range connections serve to integrate the activity of cortical nodes in brain networks. Thus, the left hemisphere might well assume different roles in neglect depending on its ability to take into account information coming from the left hemispace. "Teaching" the left hemisphere how to process ipsilateral information is a major goal of several rehabilitation techniques (see Chap. 9).

A study of resting-state functional connectivity in acute neglect patients (Carter et al. 2010) found that disruption of interhemispheric connectivity between attentional networks was correlated with impaired contralesional detection, whereas the mutual inhibition assumption of the opponent processor model would have predicted the opposite result. A functional MRI study in the monkey (Wilke et al. 2012) provided further important evidence of interhemispheric interactions in neglect-like behavior. In different trials, monkeys had either to produce saccades to peripheral targets individually presented or to choose one of two bilateral stimuli as a saccade target. Reversible pharmacological inactivation of the lateral intraparietal area resulted in a choice bias favoring ipsilesional over contralesional targets, similar to neglect/extinction behavior. Functional MRI demonstrated decreased BOLD response in nearby regions in the inactivated hemisphere for single contralesional targets. On bilateral presentations, however, when the monkey chose the contralesional target, thus countering the pharmacologically induced choice bias, there was increased activity in several frontal and parietotemporal areas in both hemispheres. These results seem in sharp contrast with the opponent processor model, which would instead have predicted increased activation for ipsilesional, not contralesional, targets in the intact hemisphere. According to Wilke et al. (2012), the bihemispheric activity pattern may indicate additional recruitment of contralesionally tuned neuronal populations because of increased effort.

6.2 Nonspatial Attention Deficits: Impaired Alertness and Sustained Attention

As described in Chap. 1, sustained attention processes have a close relationship with the functioning of right hemisphere structures. It is thus not surprising that patients with right hemisphere damage and left neglect invariably exhibit nonlateralized problems of sustained attention. For example, their manual reaction times are slowed not only for left-sided, but also for right-sided visual stimuli, albeit to a lesser extent (Bartolomeo 1997, 2001a). Moreover, their response times do not speed up with increasing time from cue to target (Bartolomeo et al. 2001a), as they typically do in normal participants (Bertelson 1967), who raise their level of vigilant attention as time passes after the appearance of the cue. Thus, as proposed by Ian Robertson, it is possible that lateralized attentional deficits are a necessary but not sufficient factor in the persistence of neglect. A second, nonspatially lateralized loss of attentional capacity must coexist with the spatial bias for the disorder to persist in a clinically substantial way (Robertson 2001). Several studies have indeed demonstrated that the degree of impairment of sustained attention is a strong predictor for the persistence of neglect (Hjaltason et al. 1996; Samuelsson et al. 1998). Consistent with this hypothesis, Robertson et al. (1998) have shown an interaction between alertness and orienting in neglect patients, suggesting that phasic alertness might affect the speed of perceptual processing in the neglected visual field. In their study, a temporal order judgment task was used, and the alerting tone speeded the processing of left-sided stimuli, overcoming patients' rightward bias of attention.

Malhotra et al. (2009) also demonstrated an interaction between sustained attention and spatial attention after right parietal damage. Neglect patients presented a vigilance decrement but only when the task involved spatial components. These vigilance decrements were associated with lesions to the PPC. Chica et al. (2012) explored neglect patients by using a response time test devised to assess three distinct attentional functions: orienting, alerting, and executive control (requiring both monitoring and conflict solving) (Fan et al. 2002; Callejas et al. 2004). In the study by Chica et al. (2012), phasic alertness triggered by an acoustic tone was able to improve the orienting deficit to left-sided targets, by reducing the interference of distractors in the neglected visual field, thus facilitating conflict resolution.

6.3 Lateralized Premotor Deficits

Visual neglect has often been considered as a disorder essentially determining an impaired *perception* of objects in space. However, perception is not the result of a passive display of the external world in the brain; on the contrary, organisms actively explore the environment in search of relevant stimuli, as stressed by the so-called active (or "animate") perception approach (Arbib 1981; Ballard 1991; Findlay and Gilchrist 2003; Miglino et al. 2009). Neglect is a case in point of this approach: patients without any elementary sensory deficits can behave as if they were completely blind to left-sided objects, because they do not explore them. Thus, lateralized deficits of motor exploration or of eye and hand motor responses may well play a major role in neglect behavior. It is important to distinguish these deficits, which are relative to the spatial position of the stimuli eliciting patients' responses, from motor neglect (described in Sect. 2.3), which is an inability to move one's contralesional limbs irrespective of the hemispace where the movement should occur.

6.3.1 Spatial Response Bias

Patients with left neglect may show a response bias when asked to press lateralized keys, even if they are close to each other, with faster responses for right-sided keys than for left-sided keys (Làdavas et al. 1994b; Behrmann et al. 1995).

Làdavas et al. (1994b, Exp. 1) asked neglect patients to respond to visual stimuli by pressing two horizontally aligned adjacent keys. Patients responded slower with the left-sided key than with the right-sided key, consistent with a response bias. In a further condition, the keyboard was reversed by 180°. Again patients were slower when pressing the key in the relative left spatial position. Another study on motor bias in neglect (Bartolomeo et al. 1998), however, reported less RT asymmetry in a relatively difficult test in which patients had to press keys situated on the left or right extremity of a computer keyboard, compared to a much easier task requiring patients to respond with a unique, centrally placed key to lateralized visual targets. Thus, at least for the neglect patients included in this study, asymmetries of responses to right- vs. left-sided visual stimuli were much larger than motor response bias.

6.3.2   Directional Hypokinesia

Directional hypokinesia is conceived as a reluctance or a slowing in performing movements towards left-sided targets. As such, it might contribute to neglect manifestations. Mesulam (1981) proposed that the premotor aspect of neglect reflects involvement of the frontal component of an attention network including also the posterior parietal and cingulate cortices and the brain stem reticular formation. Heilman et al. (1985) found that a group of six right-brain-damaged patients with left neglect were slower to initiate hand movements towards the left side of space than rightward-directed movements. Once the movement was initiated, its speed did not vary, regardless of the direction. Heilman et al. (1985) introduced the term *directional hypokinesia* to label this impairment. Their findings suggest that a motor disorder participates in neglect symptoms, but do not demonstrate whether it is a necessary component of neglect or whether it is present only in some patients. The possibly related concept of directional hypometria, i.e., insufficient amplitude of contralesionally directed movements, was originally introduced to define hypometric leftward saccades in a patient with right frontal lesion (Butter et al. 1988) and subsequently used to describe the performance of a patient showing rightward line bisection errors in the absence of other signs of left neglect (Marshall and Halligan 1995). Mattingley et al. (1992) requested brain-damaged patients to press buttons which were horizontally arranged and illuminated in sequence from left to right or in the opposite direction. Neglect patients were slower when executing leftward movements than when moving rightward. In particular, patients with retrorolandic lesions were slowed when initiating movements towards a button illuminated on the left side, whereas patients with anterior or subcortical lesions showed a decreased speed of leftward movements. Nevertheless, in this paradigm patients had to detect the occurrence (lighting) of a left-sided stimulus before moving to reach it. The confounding effect of this perceptual–attentional component might thus have added to the motor component in slowing down patients' performance.

   In another study dedicated to the premotor factors of neglect, Bisiach et al. (1985) asked 16 left neglect patients to press left- or right-sided buttons in response

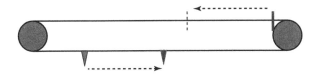

Fig. 6.5 The modified line bisection test devised by Bisiach et al. (1990) to study directional hypokinesia. The upper pointer can be moved directly or by using the bottom handle. In the latter case, the pointer is displaced in the direction opposite to the hand movement

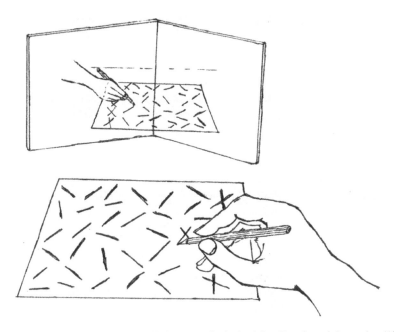

Fig. 6.6 Mirror-reversed line cancellation, a task devised by Tegnér and Levander (1991) (Redrawn from Tegnér and Levander (1991). © 1990, with permission from Oxford University Press)

to lateralized visual stimuli. Crossed and uncrossed conditions were performed, in which the side of stimulation and the side of motor response were, respectively, opposite or the same. Most errors concerned left-sided responses, irrespective of the side of stimulation. Bisiach et al. concluded that an "output neglect" was present in their patients. However, in the right stimulus/left response condition, crucial for demonstrating the output component, the ipsilesional stimulation could have captured patients' attention, thus decreasing accuracy on contralesional responses.

Other attempts to disentangle perceptual and motor aspects of neglect include a line bisection test, in which a pointer could be moved by a pulley in the direction opposite to the hand movement (Bisiach et al. 1990), (Fig. 6.5) and a line cancellation test where left and right sides could be reversed using a mirror (Fig. 6.6) (Tegnér and Levander 1991; Bisiach et al. 1995) or an epidiascope (Nico 1996).

These studies demonstrated instances of "motor" and "perceptual" forms of neglect. While perceptual factors prevailed in most neglect patients, motor factors seemed more pronounced in patients with lesions involving the frontal lobes, which appeared consistent with evidence coming from case reports (Coslett et al. 1990; Daffner et al. 1990; Bottini et al. 1992; Liu et al. 1992). However, the "motor" paradigms used in these studies were again characterized by the presence of lateralized visual feedback, thus complicating the interpretation of results. Furthermore, as noted by Mattingley and Driver (1997), the "motor" conditions in these paradigms are always more difficult to perform than the "perceptual" conditions; this may account for the tendency for patients with frontal damage to perform poorly on the "motor" conditions.

Ishiai et al. (1994a, b) adopted an easier task. They presented neglect patients with horizontal segments and asked them to extend the segment leftward to double its original length. The presence of directional hypokinesia should have reduced the length of the produced segments, but both patients with parietal lesions and patients with frontal lesions performed accurately on this task, thus not showing any signs of directional hypokinesia. Harvey et al. (1995) required eight neglect patients to point to either of the ends of a mid-transected line which they judged closer to the transection (the landmark task described in Sect. 5.3.1). Seven patients pointed consistently leftward, thus showing perceptual forms of neglect. Only one patient pointed predominantly rightward, a pattern suggestive of directional motor deficit. When Harvey and her co-workers (2002) asked 12 neglect patients to perform the epidiascope task, the pulley bisection task and the landmark test, again they observed instances of "motor" and "perceptual" forms of neglect; however, the classification of all patients except one was not consistent across the different tasks, thus raising doubts on the diagnostic validity of these procedures.

Mijovic (1991) failed to find any evidence of directional hypokinesia in a series of 40 right-brain-damaged patients who searched for a target by moving the stimulus display board under a panel until the target appeared in a window (e.g., to bring a right-sided target into view, the board was to be moved towards the left).

The conflicting results obtained in the above-reviewed studies may suggest that a directional motor disorder is a comparatively rare phenomenon in neglect or that the employed tasks did not always suitably disclose this deficit. As mentioned in the previous section, Bartolomeo et al. (1998) tried to disentangle the relative contribution of perceptual and motor factors by using two RT tasks: a perceptual task, characterized by lateralized visual stimuli and central motor responses, and a motor task, consisting of central visual stimuli and lateralized motor responses. Stimuli were arranges as a horizontal or a vertical traffic light, respectively (Bartolomeo 2002). Neglect patients showed a substantial rightward bias on the perceptual task, but only two patients (showing no signs of severe neglect) were consistently slowed in producing leftward motor responses. Bartolomeo et al. (1998) concluded that different reference frames are used in perceptual tasks and tasks involving lateralized arm movements and that visual neglect commonly results from attention disorders operating upon visual perceptual frames of reference; additional deficits, not necessarily present in all neglect patients, appear to be necessary to produce a directional motor disorder (see also Coulthard et al. 2007). Further work by Rossit et al. (2009) confirmed that manual pointing and reaching deficits are rare in neglect patients and likely to result from damage to networks partially different from those typically associated with neglect (see also Sapir et al. 2007, and Chap. 7).

6.4 Spatially Nonlateralized Deficits

6.4.1 Impaired Spatial Working Memory

Over and above their impaired spatial exploration, neglect patients may show deficits of short-term visual memory for left-sided items (D'Erme and Bartolomeo 1997). However, nonlateralized deficits of spatial working memory (SWM) may also contribute to the clinical picture. Husain and co-workers (Husain et al. 2001; Wojciulik et al. 2001, 2004; Malhotra et al. 2005) suggested that such a nonlateral-ized SWM impairment may exacerbate neglect, by impairing patients' ability to keep track of spatial locations (see also Pisella and Mattingley 2004). In cancellation tests, impaired SWM would cause patients to revisit previously detected targets and to treat them as if they had not been seen before. Consistent with this hypothesis, patients' neglect in cancellation tasks increased when targets did not change their appearance after having been touched (Husain et al. 2001; Wojciulik et al. 2001), a condition particularly taxing for SWM because there is no external cue indicating that a target has already been explored.

To further explore the SWM deficit, Mannan et al. (2005) asked 16 neglect patients to perform a computerized search task, where they had to click on newly found items while their eye movements were tracked. Clicking did not induce any modifications on found targets. Thus, "re-clicking" on previously found targets indicated that patients erroneously responded to these as new discoveries. Ten patients, with damage involving the right IPS, the right inferior frontal lobe, or both, tended to re-click on previously found targets on the right at a pathological rate. Increased re-clicking with time interval between the first and the second click was associated with parietal damage, whereas flat re-click functions were associated with frontal/subcortical lesions. Thus, two different mechanisms might underlie re-clicking behavior in neglect patients: a failure to keep track of spatial locations during search in parietal patients or a deficit of response inhibition ("perseverative" behavior) in patients with more anterior lesions. However, none of the re-clicking patients showed perseverative behavior on paper-and-pencil cancellation tests (Na et al. 1999; Rusconi et al. 2002), and one patient who perseverated in cancelling right-sided items on standard tests did not re-click on the computerized task.

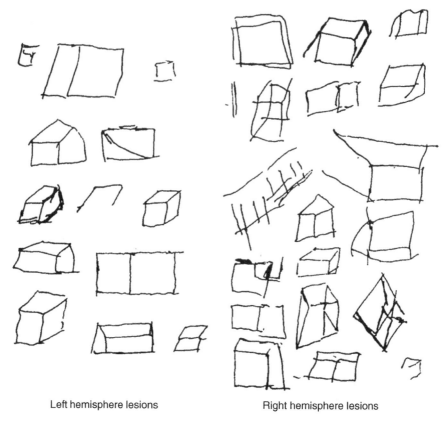

Left hemisphere lesions   Right hemisphere lesions

Fig. 6.7 Copies of a cube made by patients with left or right hemisphere lesions (Reproduced from Piercy et al. (1960). © 1960, with permission from Oxford University Press)

6.4.2 Constructional Apraxia

The term constructional apraxia refers to the patients' inability to make an accurate copy of two-dimensional drawings or three-dimensional objects, in the absence of apraxic deficits for single movements (Kleist 1934). Constructional apraxia can thus be characterized by impaired assembling of multipart objects. Patients with right hemisphere damage may show lack of accurate spatial organization in their graphic production, with details transposed to different spatial positions or orientations. These problems are not necessarily lateralized to the left side of the drawing and may persist after lateralized sings of neglect have resolved (Hier et al. 1983). Patients with left hemisphere damage may also show signs of constructional apraxia, but with different characteristics, such as oversimplified and reduced productions (Gainotti and Tiacci 1970) (Fig. 6.7).

Pisella and Mattingley (2004) have suggested that visual information is integrated across fixations thanks to processes of spatial remapping implemented in the parietal lobes (Duhamel et al. 1992), with a right hemisphere dominance in humans (Pisella et al. 2011). A failure of these remapping processes may account for some neglect-related phenomena, such as mislocations of left-sided details, as seen in allochiria (see Sect. 4.5.1), in extinction (see Sect. 2.2), or in constructional apraxia. Consistent with this hypothesis, Vuilleumier et al. (2007) demonstrated that patients with left neglect had a dramatic loss of memory for target location after shifting their gaze to its right, so that the target was now to the left of fixation. Russel et al. (2010) found a tight link between impaired remapping of spatial information across saccadic eye movements and clinical signs of constructional apraxia in right-hemisphere stroke patients.

6.5   Imaginal Deficits

As mentioned in Sect. 4.6, patients may show signs of neglect even when they are not directly interacting with their environment. In this case, patients seem to ignore the left half of their internal images. These forms of "representational" or imaginal neglect are however much rarer than the typical "perceptual" forms (see Bartolomeo et al. 1994, Sect. 4.6 and 5.4.3). In one study (Bartolomeo et al. 1994), imaginal neglect was present in only one third of patients with visuospatial neglect; however, the scores for the two forms of neglect showed a linear relationship, suggesting some common mechanism. Despite this, the typical tendency to start the visuospatial tests from the rightmost item, consistent with the magnetic attraction phenomenon, was present for the visuospatial tasks but absent for the imaginal tasks. This finding confirms that imaginal neglect has a status of its own, whose possible contributions to visuospatial signs remain uncertain.

6.6   Impaired Processing of Time

Patients with neglect do not only show deficits of spatial cognition but also impaired processing of temporal information. Basso et al. (1996) described a right-brain-damaged patient who consistently overestimated the duration of stimuli presented in the neglected space, for temporal intervals in the hundreds of milliseconds range. Harrington et al. (1998) found evidence for impaired time perception within a similar temporal range in patients with right hemispheric damage, but not in left-brain-damaged patients. These deficits were present in patients with frontoparietal lesions and correlated with impaired performance on a test of nonspatial attention. Danckert et al. (2007) demonstrated that neglect patients grossly underestimated multi-second temporal durations. These results are not surprising, given that focusing attention on temporal intervals relies on brain networks partly overlapping with those of spatial orienting, including PPC (Eagleman et al. 2005) and PFC (Triviño et al. 2010). A cortical "when" pathway for temporal processing has also been proposed in the right hemisphere (Battelli et al. 2007), going from the visual occipital areas to the right TPJ through the middle temporal area specialized with movement processing. More generally, the parietal cortex may have a special role in the processing of magnitudes, including time, space, and numbers (Bueti and Walsh 2009).

References

Anderson B, Mennemeier M, Chatterjee A. Variability not ability: another basis for performance decrements in neglect. Neuropsychologia. 2000;38:785–96.

Arbib MA. Perceptual structures and distributed motor control. In: Brooks VB, editor. Handbook of physiology: the nervous system II. Motor control. Bethesda: American Physiological Society; 1981. p. 1449–80.

Ballard DH. Animate vision. Artif Intell. 1991;48:57–86.

Bartolomeo P. The novelty effect in recovered hemineglect. Cortex. 1997;33:323–32.

Bartolomeo P. The traffic light paradigm: a reaction time task to study laterally directed arm movements. Brain Res Brain Res Protoc. 2002;9:32–40.

Bartolomeo P. Visual neglect. Curr Opin Neurol. 2007;20:381–6.

Bartolomeo P, Chokron S. Left unilateral neglect or right hyperattention? Neurology. 1999;53:2023–7.

Bartolomeo P, Chokron S. Levels of impairment in unilateral neglect. In: Boller F, Grafman J, editors. Handbook of neuropsychology. 2nd ed. Amsterdam: Elsevier Science Publishers; 2001. p. 67–98.

Bartolomeo P, Chokron S. Orienting of attention in left unilateral neglect. Neurosci Biobehav Rev. 2002;26:217–34.

Bartolomeo P, D'Erme P, Gainotti G. The relationship between visuospatial and representational neglect. Neurology. 1994;44:1710–4.

Bartolomeo P, D'Erme P, Perri R, Gainotti G. Perception and action in hemispatial neglect. Neuropsychologia. 1998;36:227–37.

Bartolomeo P, Chokron S, Siéroff E. Facilitation instead of inhibition for repeated right-sided events in left neglect. Neuroreport. 1999;10:3353–7.

Bartolomeo P, Siéroff E, Decaix C, Chokron S. Modulating the attentional bias in unilateral neglect: the effects of the strategic set. Exp Brain Res. 2001a;137:424–31.

Bartolomeo P, Siéroff E, Chokron S, Decaix C. Variability of response times as a marker of diverted attention. Neuropsychologia. 2001b;39:358–63.

Bartolomeo P, Urbanski M, Chokron S, Chainay H, Moroni C, Siéroff E, Belin C, Halligan P. Neglected attention in apparent spatial compression. Neuropsychologia. 2004;42:49–61.

Bartolomeo P, Thiebaut de Schotten M, Doricchi F. Left unilateral neglect as a disconnection syndrome. Cereb Cortex. 2007;45:3127–48.

Barton JJ, Behrmann M, Black S. Ocular search during line bisection. The effects of hemi-neglect and hemianopia. Brain. 1998;121:1117–31.

Basso G, Nichelli P, Frassinetti F, di Pellegrino G. Time perception in a neglected space. Neuroreport. 1996;7:2111–4.

Battelli L, Pascual-Leone A, Cavanagh P. The 'when' pathway of the right parietal lobe. Trends Cogn Sci. 2007;11:204–10.

Behrmann M, Moscovitch M. Object-centered neglect in patients with unilateral neglect: effects of left-right coordinates of objects. J Cogn Neurosci. 1994;6:1–16.

Behrmann M, Tipper SP. Attention accesses multiple reference frames: evidence from visual neglect. J Exp Psychol Hum Percept Perform. 1999;25:83–101.

Behrmann M, Black SE, Murji S. Spatial attention in the mental architecture: evidence from neuropsychology. J Clin Exp Neuropsychol. 1995;17:220–42.

Bertelson P. The time course of prepration. Q J Exp Psychol. 1967;19:272–9.

Berti A, Frassinetti F, Umiltà C. Nonconscious reading? Evidence from neglect dyslexia. Cortex. 1994;30:181–97.

Bisiach E. Mental representation in unilateral neglect and related disorders. Q J Exp Psychol. 1993;46A:435–61.

Bisiach E, Berti A, Vallar G. Analogical and logical disorders underlying unilateral neglect of space. In: Posner MI, Marin OS, editors. Attention and performance XI. Hillsdale: Lawrence Erlbaum Associates; 1985. p. 239–49.

Bisiach E, Geminiani G, Berti A, Rusconi ML. Perceptual and premotor factors of unilateral neglect. Neurology. 1990;40:1278–81.

Bisiach E, Rusconi ML, Peretti VA, Vallar G. Challenging current accounts of unilateral neglect. Neuropsychologia. 1994;32:1431–4.

Bisiach E, Tegnér R, Làdavas E, Rusconi ML, Mijovic' D, Hjaltason H. Dissociation of ophtalmo-kinetic and melokinetic attention in unilateral neglect. Cereb Cortex. 1995;5:439–47.

Boly M, Balteau E, Schnakers C, Degueldre C, Moonen G, Luxen A, Phillips C, Peigneux P, Maquet P, Laureys S. Baseline brain activity fluctuations predict somatosensory perception in humans. Proc Natl Acad Sci. 2007;104:12187–92.

Bottini G, Sterzi R, Vallar G. Directional hypokinesia in spatial hemineglect: a case study. J Neurol Neurosurg Psychiatry. 1992;55:562–5.

Bourgeois A, Chica AB, Migliaccio R, Thiebaut de Schotten M, Bartolomeo P. Cortical control of inhibition of return: evidence from patients with inferior parietal damage and visual neglect. Neuropsychologia. 2012;50:800–9.

Bourgeois A, Chica AB, Valero-Cabré A, Bartolomeo P. Cortical control of inhibition of return: causal evidence for task-dependent modulations by dorsal and ventral parietal regions. Cortex. 2013a;49:2229–38.

Bourgeois A, Chica AB, Valero-Cabré A, Bartolomeo P. Cortical control of inhibition of return: exploring the causal contributions of the left parietal cortex. Cortex. 2013b; doi: 10.1016/j. cortex.2013.08.004. [Epub ahead of print]

Bueti D, Walsh V. The parietal cortex and the representation of time, space, number and other magnitudes. Philos Trans R Soc Lond B Biol Sci. 2009;364:1831–40.

Buschman TJ, Miller EK. Top-down versus bottom-up control of attention in the prefrontal and posterior parietal cortices. Science. 2007;315:1860–2.

Butter CM, Rapcsak S, Watson RT, Heilman KM. Changes in sensory inattention, directional motor neglect and "release" of the fixation reflex following a unilateral frontal lesion: a case report. Neuropsychologia. 1988;26:533–45.

Callejas A, Lupiáñez J, Tudela P. The three attentional networks: on their independence and interactions. Brain Cogn. 2004;54:225–7.

Caramazza A, Hillis AE. Spatial representation of words in the brain implied by studies of a unilateral neglect patient. Nature. 1990;346:267–9.

Carter AR, Astafiev SV, Lang CE, Connor LT, Rengachary J, Strube MJ, Pope DLW, Shulman GL, Corbetta M. Resting interhemispheric functional magnetic resonance imaging connectivity predicts performance after stroke. Ann Neurol. 2010;67:365–75.

Chica AB, Lasaponara S, Lupiáñez J, Doricchi F, Bartolomeo P. Exogenous attention can capture perceptual consciousness: ERP and behavioural evidence. Neuroimage. 2010;51:1205–12.

Chica AB, Bartolomeo P, Valero-Cabre A. Dorsal and ventral parietal contributions to spatial orienting in the human brain. J Neurosci. 2011a;31:8143–9.

Chica AB, Lasaponara S, Chanes L, Valero-Cabré A, Doricchi F, Lupiáñez J, Bartolomeo P. Spatial attention and conscious perception: the role of endogenous and exogenous orienting. Atten Percept Psychophys. 2011b;73:1065–81.

Chica AB, Thiebaut de Schotten M, Toba MN, Malhotra P, Lupiáñez J, Bartolomeo P. Attention networks and their interactions after right-hemisphere damage. Cortex. 2012;48:654–63.

Corbetta M, Kincade MJ, Lewis C, Snyder AZ, Sapir A. Neural basis and recovery of spatial attention deficits in spatial neglect. Nat Neurosci. 2005;8:1603–10.

Coslett HB, Bowers D, Fitzpatrick E, Haws B, Heilman KM. Directional hypokinesia and hemispatial inattention in neglect. Brain. 1990;113:475–86.

Coulthard E, Parton A, Husain M. The modular architecture of the neglect syndrome: implications for action control in visual neglect. Neuropsychologia. 2007;45:1982–4.

D'Erme P, Bartolomeo P. A unilateral defect of short-term visual memory in left hemineglect. Eur J Neurol. 1997;4:382–6.

D'Erme P, Robertson I, Bartolomeo P, Daniele A, Gainotti G. Early rightwards orienting of attention on simple reaction time performance in patients with left-sided neglect. Neuropsychologia. 1992;30:989–1000.

D'Erme P, Robertson IH, Bartolomeo P, Daniele A. Unilateral neglect: the fate of the extinguished visual stimuli. Behav Neurol. 1993;6:143–50.

Daffner KR, Ahern GL, Weintraub S, Mesulam M-M. Dissociated neglect behaviour following sequential strokes in the right hemisphere. Ann Neurol. 1990;28:97–101.

Danckert J, Ferber S, Pun C, Broderick C, Striemer C, Rock S, Stewart D. Neglected time: impaired temporal perception of multisecond intervals in unilateral neglect. J Cogn Neurosci. 2007;19:1706–20.

Doricchi F, Incoccia C, Galati G. Influence of figure-ground contrast on the implicit and explicit processing of line drawings in patients with left unilateral neglect. Cogn Neuropsychol. 1997;14:573–94.

Dorris MC, Klein RM, Everling S, Munoz DP. Contribution of the primate superior colliculus to inhibition of return. J Cogn Neurosci. 2002;14:1256–63.

Doty R. Forebrain commissures: glimpses of neurons producing mind. In: Zaidel E, Iacoboni M, editors. The parallel brain: the cognitive neuroscience of the corpus callosum. Cambridge, MA: The MIT Press; 2003. p. 157–65.

Driver J, Halligan PW. Can visual neglect operate in object-centered co-ordinates? An affirmative single-case study. Cogn Neuropsychol. 1991;8:475–96.

Driver J, Pouget A. Object-centered visual neglect, or relative egocentric neglect? J Cogn Neurosci. 2000;12:542–5.

Driver J, Baylis GC, Goodrich SJ, Rafal RD. Axis-based neglect of visual shapes. Neuropsychologia. 1994;32:1353–65.

Duhamel JR, Colby CL, Goldberg ME. The updating of the representation of visual space in parietal cortex by intended eye movements. Science. 1992;255:90–2.

Eagleman DM, Tse PU, Buonomano D, Janssen P, Nobre AC, Holcombe AO. Time and the brain: how subjective time relates to neural time. J Neurosci. 2005;25:10369–71.

Egly R, Driver J, Rafal RD. Shifting visual attention between objects and locations: evidence from normal and parietal lesion patients. J Exp Psychol Gen. 1994;123:161–77.

Fan J, McCandliss BD, Sommer T, Raz A, Posner MI. Testing the efficiency and independence of attentional networks. J Cogn Neurosci. 2002;14:340–7.

Farah MJ, Brunn JL, Wong AB, Wallace MA, Carpenter PA. Frames of reference for allocating attention to space: evidence from the neglect syndrome. Neuropsychologia. 1990;28:335–47.

Findlay JM, Gilchrist ID. Active vision: the psychology of looking and seeing. Oxford: Oxford University Press; 2003.

Fox MD, Raichle ME. Spontaneous fluctuations in brain activity observed with functional magnetic resonance imaging. Nat Rev Neurosci. 2007;8:700–11.

Gainotti G, Tiacci C. Patterns of drawing disability in right and left hemispheric patients. Neuropsychologia. 1970;8:379–84.

Gainotti G, Messerli P, Tissot R. Qualitative analysis of unilateral spatial neglect in relation to the laterality of cerebral lesions. J Neurol Neurosurg Psychiatry. 1972;35:545–50.

Gainotti G, D'Erme P, Bartolomeo P. Early orientation of attention toward the half space ipsilateral to the lesion in patients with unilateral brain damage. J Neurol Neurosurg Psychiatry. 1991;54:1082–9.

Gainotti G, Bourlon C, Bartolomeo P. La négligence spatiale unilatérale. In: Lechevalier B, Viader F, Eustache F, editors. Traité de neuropsychologie clinique. Bruxelles/Paris: De Boeck – Inserm; 2008. p. 627–49.

Gazzaniga MS, Baynes K. Consciousness, introspection, and the split-brain: the two minds/one body problem. In: Gazzaniga MS, editor. The new cognitive neurosciences. Cambridge, MA: MIT Press; 2000. p. 1355–63.

Geschwind N. Disconnexion syndromes in animals and man – part II. Brain. 1965;88:585–644.

Gross J, Schmitz F, Schnitzler I, Kessler K, Shapiro K, Hommel B, Schnitzler A. Modulation of long-range neural synchrony reflects temporal limitations of visual attention in humans. Proc Natl Acad Sci U S A. 2004;101:13050–5.

Habekost T, Rostrup E. Visual attention capacity after right hemisphere lesions. Neuropsychologia. 2007;45:1474–88.

Harrington DL, Haaland KY, Knight RT. Cortical networks underlying mechanisms of time perception. J Neurosci. 1998;18:1085–95.

Harvey M, Milner AD, Roberts RC. An investigation of hemispatial neglect using the landmark task. Brain Cogn. 1995;27:59–78.

Harvey M, Kramer-McCaffery T, Dow L, Murphy PJ, Gilchrist ID. Categorisation of 'perceptual' and 'premotor' neglect patients across different tasks: is there strong evidence for a dichotomy? Neuropsychologia. 2002;40:1387–95.

Heilman KM, Bowers D, Coslett HB, Whelan H, Watson RT. Directional hypokinesia: prolonged reaction times for leftward movements in patients with right hemisphere lesions and neglect. Neurology. 1985;35:855–9.

Hier DB, Mondlock J, Caplan LR. Recovery of behavioral abnormalities after right hemisphere stroke. Neurology. 1983;33:345–50.

Hjaltason H, Tegner R, Tham K, Levander M, Ericson K. Sustained attention and awareness of disability in chronic neglect. Neuropsychologia. 1996;34:1229–33.

Husain M, Rorden C. Non-spatially lateralized mechanisms in hemispatial neglect. Nat Rev Neurosci. 2003;4:26–36.

Husain M, Shapiro K, Martin J, Kennard C. Abnormal temporal dynamics of visual attention in spatial neglect patients. Nature. 1997;385:154–6.

Husain M, Mannan S, Hodgson T, Wojciulik E, Driver J, Kennard C. Impaired spatial working memory across saccades contributes to abnormal search in parietal neglect. Brain. 2001;124:941–52.

Ishiai S, Watabiki S, Lee E, Kanouchi T, Odajima N. Preserved leftward movement in left unilateral spatial neglect due to frontal lesions. J Neurol Neurosurg Psychiatry. 1994a;57: 1085–90.

Ishiai S, Sugushita M, Watabiki S, Nakayama T, Kotera M, Gono S. Improvement of left unilateral spatial neglect in a line extension task. Neurology. 1994b;44:294–8.

Ishiai S, Seki K, Koyama Y, Gono S. Ineffective leftward search in line bisection and mechanisms of left unilateral spatial neglect. J Neurol. 1996;243:381–7.

Kinsbourne M. Orientational bias model of unilateral neglect: evidence from attentional gradients within hemispace. In: Robertson IH, Marshall JC, editors. Unilateral neglect: clinical and experimental studies. Hove: Lawrence Erlbaum Associates; 1993. p. 63–86.

Kleist K. Gehirnpathologie. Leipzig: Barth; 1934.

Koch G, Oliveri M, Cheeran B, Ruge D, Lo Gerfo E, Salerno S, Torriero S, Marconi B, Mori F, Driver J, Rothwell JC, Caltagirone C. Hyperexcitability of parietal-motor functional connections in the intact left-hemisphere of patients with neglect. Brain. 2008;131:3147–55.

Làdavas E, Carletti M, Gori G. Automatic and voluntary orienting of attention in patients with visual neglect: horizontal and vertical dimensions. Neuropsychologia. 1994a;32:1195–208.

Làdavas E, Farne A, Carletti M, Zeloni G. Neglect determined by the relative location of responses. Brain. 1994b;117:705–14.

Làdavas E, Zeloni G, Zaccara G, Gangemi P. Eye movements and orienting of attention in patients with visual neglect. J Cogn Neurosci. 1997;9:67–74.

Liu GT, Bolton AR, Price BH, Weintraub S. Dissociated perceptual-sensory and exploratory-motor neglect. J Neurol Neurosurg Psychiatry. 1992;55:701–6.

Losier BJ, Klein RM. A review of the evidence for a disengage deficit following parietal lobe damage. Neurosci Biobehav Rev. 2001;25:1–13.

Lupiáñez J, Decaix C, Siéroff E, Chokron S, Milliken B, Bartolomeo P. Independent effects of endogenous and exogenous spatial cueing: inhibition of return at endogenously attended target locations. Exp Brain Res. 2004;159:447–57.

Macquistan AD. Object-based allocation of visual attention in response to exogenous, but not endogenous, spatial precues. Psychon Bull Rev. 1997;4:512–5.

Malhotra P, Jager HR, Parton A, Greenwood R, Playford ED, Brown MM, Driver J, Husain M. Spatial working memory capacity in unilateral neglect. Brain. 2005;128:424–35.

Malhotra P, Coulthard EJ, Husain M. Role of right posterior parietal cortex in maintaining attention to spatial locations over time. Brain. 2009;132:645–60.

Mannan SK, Mort DJ, Hodgson TL, Driver J, Kennard C, Husain M. Revisiting previously searched locations in visual neglect: role of right parietal and frontal lesions in misjudging old locations as new. J Cogn Neurosci. 2005;17:340–54.

Manning L, Kartsounis LD. Confabulations related to tacit awareness in visual neglect. Behav Neurol. 1993;6:211–3.

Marshall JC, Halligan PW. Blindsight and insight into visuo-spatial neglect. Nature. 1988; 336:766–7.

Marshall JC, Halligan P. Within- and between-task dissociations in visuo-spatial neglect: a case study. Cortex. 1995;31:367–76.

Mattingley JB, Driver J. Distinguishing sensory and motor deficits after parietal damage: an evaluation of reponse selection biases in unilateral neglect. In: Thier P, Karnath HO, editors. Parietal lobe contributions to orientation in 3D-space. Heidelberg: Springer; 1997. p. 309–37.

Mattingley JB, Bradshaw JL, Phillips JG. Impairments of movement initiation and execution in unilateral neglect. Brain. 1992;115:1849–74.

Mattingley JB, Bradshaw JL, Bradshaw JA, Nettleton NC. Residual rightward attentional bias after apparent recovery from right hemisphere damage: implications for a multicomponent model of neglect. J Neurol Neurosurg Psychiatry. 1994;57:597–604.

McGlinchey-Berroth R, Milberg W, Verfaellie M, Alexander M, Kiduff PT. Semantic processing in the neglected visual field: evidence from a lexical decision task. Cogn Neuropsychol. 1993;10:79–108.

Mesulam MM. A cortical network for directed attention and unilateral neglect. Ann Neurol. 1981;10:309–25.

Miceli G, Capasso R. Word-centred neglect dyslexia: evidence from a new case. Neurocase. 2001;7:221–3.

Miglino O, Ponticorvo M, Bartolomeo P. Place cognition and active perception: a study with evolved robots. Connect Sci. 2009;21:3–14.

Mijovic' D. Mechanisms of visual spatial neglect: absence of directional hypokinesia in spatial exploration. Brain. 1991;114:1575–93.

Morrow LA, Ratcliff G. The disengagement of covert attention and the neglect syndrome. Psychobiology. 1988;16:261–9.

Müller HJ, Findlay JM. The effect of visual attention on peripheral discrimination thresholds in single and multiple element displays. Acta Psychol (Amst). 1988;69:129–55.

Müller HJ, Rabbitt PM. Reflexive and voluntary orienting of visual attention: time course of activation and resistance to interruption. J Exp Psychol Hum Percept Perform. 1989;15:315–30.

Na DL, Adair JC, Kang Y, Chung CS, Lee KH, Heilman KM. Motor perseverative behavior on a line cancellation task. Neurology. 1999;52:1569–76.

Nakayama K, Mackeben M. Sustained and transient components of focal visual attention. Vision Res. 1989;29:1631–47.

Natale E, Marzi CA, Bricolo E, Johannsen L, Karnath HO. Abnormally speeded saccades to ipsilesional targets in patients with spatial neglect. Neuropsychologia. 2007;45:263–72.

Nico D. Detecting directional hypokinesia: the epidiascope technique. Neuropsychologia. 1996;34:471–4.

Oliveri M, Rossini PM, Traversa R, Cicinelli P, Filippi MM, Pasqualetti P, Tomaiuolo F, Caltagirone C. Left frontal transcranial magnetic stimulation reduces contralesional extinction in patients with unilateral right brain damage. Brain. 1999;122(Pt 9):1731–9.

Ota H, Fujii T, Suzuki K, Fukatsu R, Yamadori A. Dissociation of body-centered and stimulus-centered representations in unilateral neglect. Neurology. 2001;57:2064–2069.

Pantano P, Di Piero V, Fieschi C, Judica A, Guariglia C, Pizzamiglio L. Pattern of CBF in the rehabilitation of visual spatial neglect. Int J Neurosci. 1992;66:153–61.

Perani D, Vallar G, Paulesu E, Alberoni M, Fazio F. Left and right hemisphere contribution to recovery from neglect after right hemisphere damage – An [18F]FDG PET study of two cases. Neuropsychologia. 1993;31:115–25.

Piercy M, Hécaen H, de Ajuriaguerra J. Constructional apraxia associated with unilateral cerebral lesions – left and right sided cases compared. Brain. 1960;83:225–42.

Pisella L, Mattingley JB. The contribution of spatial remapping impairments to unilateral visual neglect. Neurosci Biobehav Rev. 2004;28:181–200.

Pisella L, Alahyane N, Blangero A, Thery F, Blanc S, Pelisson D. Right-hemispheric dominance for visual remapping in humans. Philos Trans R Soc Lond B Biol Sci. 2011;366:572–85.

Posner MI. Orienting of attention. Q J Exp Psychol. 1980;32:3–25.

Posner MI, Cohen Y, Rafal RD. Neural systems control of spatial orienting. Philos Trans R Soc Lond B Biol Sci. 1982;298:187–98.

Posner MI, Walker JA, Friedrich FJ, Rafal RD. Effects of parietal injury on covert orienting of attention. J Neurosci. 1984;4:1863–74.

Posner MI, Walker JA, Friedrich FA, Rafal RD. How do the parietal lobes direct covert attention? Neuropsychologia. 1987;25:135–45.

Pratt J, McAuliffe J. The effects of onsets and offsets on visual attention. Psychol Res. 2001;65:185–91.

Rafal RD, Posner MI, Friedman JH, Inhoff AW, Bernstein E. Orienting of visual attention in progressive supranuclear palsy. Brain. 1988;111:267–80.

Rafal RD, Calabresi PA, Brennan CW, Sciolto TK. Saccade preparation inhibits reorienting to recently attended locations. J Exp Psychol Hum Percept Perform. 1989;15:673–85.

Rastelli F, Funes MJ, Lupiáñez J, Duret C, Bartolomeo P. Left neglect: is the disengage deficit space- or object-based? Exp Brain Res. 2008;187:439–46.

Rastelli F, Tallon-Baudry C, Migliaccio R, Toba MN, Ducorps A, Pradat-Diehl P, Duret C, Dubois B, Valero-Cabré A, Bartolomeo P. Neural dynamics of neglected targets in patients with right hemisphere damage. Cortex. 2013;49:1989–96.

Ress D, Backus BT, Heeger DJ. Activity in primary visual cortex predicts performance in a visual detection task. Nat Neurosci. 2000;3:940–5.

Riggio L, Kirsner K. The relationship between central cues and peripheral cues in covert visual orientation. Percept Psychophys. 1997;59:885–99.

Ro T, Farné A, Chang E. Inhibition of return and the human frontal eye fields. Exp Brain Res. 2003;150:290–6.

Robertson IH. Do we need the "lateral" in unilateral neglect? Spatially nonselective attention deficits in unilateral neglect and their implications for rehabilitation. Neuroimage. 2001;14:S85–90.

Robertson IH, Mattingley JB, Rorden C, Driver J. Phasic alerting of neglect patients overcomes their spatial deficit in visual awareness. Nature. 1998;395:169–72.

Rossit S, Malhotra P, Muir K, Reeves I, Duncan G, Livingstone K, Jackson H, Hogg C, Castle P, Learmonth G, Harvey M. No neglect-specific deficits in reaching tasks. Cereb Cortex. 2009;19:2616–24.

Rusconi ML, Maravita A, Bottini G, Vallar G. Is the intact side really intact? Perseverative responses in patients with unilateral neglect: a productive manifestation. Neuropsychologia. 2002;40:594–604.

Rushmore RJ, Valero-Cabre A, Lomber SG, Hilgetag CC, Payne BR. Functional circuitry underlying visual neglect. Brain. 2006;129:1803–21.

Russell C, Deidda C, Malhotra P, Crinion JT, Merola S, Husain M. A deficit of spatial remapping in constructional apraxia after right-hemisphere stroke. Brain. 2010;133:1239–51.

Samuelsson H, Hjelmquist EK, Jensen C, Ekholm S, Blomstrand C. Nonlateralized attentional deficits: an important component behind persisting visuospatial neglect? J Clin Exp Neuropsychol. 1998;20:73–88.

Sapir A, Soroker N, Berger A, Henik A. Inhibition of return in spatial attention: direct evidence for collicular generation. Nat Neurosci. 1999;2:1053–4.

Sapir A, Kaplan JB, He BJ, Corbetta M. Anatomical correlates of directional hypokinesia in patients with hemispatial neglect. J Neurosci. 2007;27:4045–51.

Seki K, Ishiai S, Koyama Y, Fujimoto Y. Appearance and disappearance of unilateral spatial neglect for an object: influence of attention-attracting peripheral stimuli. Neuropsychologia. 1996;34:819–26.

Shepherd M, Findlay JM, Hockey RJ. The relationship between eye movements and spatial attention. Q J Exp Psychol. 1986;38A:475–791.

Siéroff E, Decaix C, Chokron S, Bartolomeo P. Impaired orienting of attention in left unilateral neglect: a componential analysis. Neuropsychology. 2007;21:94–113.

Small M, Ellis S. Brief remission periods in visuospatial neglect: evidence from long-term follow-up. Eur Neurol. 1994;34:147–54.

Smania N, Martini MC, Gambina G, Tomelleri G, Palamara A, Natale E, Marzi CA. The spatial distribution of visual attention in hemineglect and extinction patients. Brain. 1998;121:1759–70.

Snow JC, Mattingley JB. Goal-driven selective attention in patients with right hemisphere lesions: how intact is the ipsilesional field? Brain. 2006;129:168–81.

Sprague JM. Interaction of cortex and superior colliculus in mediation of visually guided behavior in the cat. Science. 1966;153:1544–7.

Striemer C, Danckert J. Prism adaptation reduces the disengage deficit in right brain damage patients. Neuroreport. 2007;18:99–103.

Tegnér R, Levander M. Through a looking glass. A new technique to demonstrate directional hypokinesia in unilateral neglect. Brain. 1991;114:1943–51.

Triviño M, Correa A, Arnedo M, Lupiáñez J. Temporal orienting deficit after prefrontal damage. Brain. 2010;133:1173–85.

Valdes-Sosa M, Bobes MA, Rodriguez V, Pinilla T. Switching attention without shifting the spotlight object-based attentional modulation of brain potentials. J Cogn Neurosci. 1998;10:137–51.

Vivas AB, Humphreys GW, Fuentes LJ. Inhibitory processing following damage to the parietal lobe. Neuropsychologia. 2003;41:1531–40.

Vivas AB, Humphreys GW, Fuentes LJ. Abnormal inhibition of return: a review and new data on patients with parietal lobe damage. Cogn Neuropsychol. 2006;23:1049–64.

Volpe BT, Ledoux JE, Gazzaniga MS. Information processing of visual stimuli in an "extinguished" field. Nature. 1979;282:722–4.

Vuilleumier P, Hester D, Assal G, Regli F. Unilateral spatial neglect recovery after sequential strokes. Neurology. 1996;46:184–9.

Vuilleumier P, Sagiv N, Hazeltine E, Poldrack RA, Swick D, Rafal RD, Gabrieli JD. Neural fate of seen and unseen faces in visuospatial neglect: a combined event-related functional MRI and event-related potential study. Proc Natl Acad Sci U S A. 2001;98:3495–500.

Vuilleumier P, Sergent C, Schwartz S, Valenza N, Girardi M, Husain M, Driver J. Impaired perceptual memory of locations across gaze-shifts in patients with unilateral spatial neglect. J Cogn Neurosci. 2007;19:1388–406.

Wade DT, Wood VA, Hewer RL. Recovery of cognitive function soon after stroke: a study of visual neglect, attention span and verbal recall. J Neurol Neurosurg Psychiatry. 1988; 51:10–3.

Wilke M, Kagan I, Andersen RA. Functional imaging reveals rapid reorganization of cortical activity after parietal inactivation in monkeys. Proc Natl Acad Sci. 2012;109:8274–9.

Wojciulik E, Husain M, Clarke K, Driver J. Spatial working memory deficit in unilateral neglect. Neuropsychologia. 2001;39:390–6.

Wojciulik E, Rorden C, Clarke K, Husain M, Driver J. Group study of an "undercover" test for visuospatial neglect: invisible cancellation can reveal more neglect than standard cancellation. J Neurol Neurosurg Psychiatry. 2004;75:1356–8.

Yantis S, Jonides J. Abrupt visual onsets and selective attention: voluntary versus automatic allocation. J Exp Psychol Hum Percept Perform. 1990;16:121–34.

Further Reading

Coulthard E, Parton A, Husain M. The modular architecture of the neglect syndrome: implications for action control in visual neglect. Neuropsychologia. 2007;45(8):1982–4.

Danckert J. Spatial neglect: not simply disordered attention. In: Schweizer TA, Macdonald RL, editors. The behavioral consequences of stroke. New York: Springer; 2013. p. 71–94.

Husain M, Rorden C. Non-spatially lateralized mechanisms in hemispatial neglect. Nat Rev Neurosci. 2003;4(1):26–36.

Losier BJ, Klein RM. A review of the evidence for a disengage deficit following parietal lobe damage. Neurosci Biobehav Rev. 2001;25(1):1–13.

Pisella L, Mattingley JB. The contribution of spatial remapping impairments to unilateral visual neglect. Neurosci Biobehav Rev. 2004;28(2):181–200.

Robertson IH. Do we need the "lateral" in unilateral neglect? Spatially nonselective attention deficits in unilateral neglect and their implications for rehabilitation. Neuroimage. 2001;14(1):S85–90.

Chapter 7
The Anatomy of Neglect

Keywords Parietal lobe • Temporal lobe • Frontal lobe • Occipital lobe • Basal ganglia • Thalamus • Superior longitudinal fasciculus • Inferior fronto-occipital fasciculus

A central problem in cognitive neurology concerns the manner of relating neural structure and circuit functioning to cognitive performance. Paul Broca's description of his patient Leborgne, who suffered from vascular damage to the inferior frontal lobe of the left hemisphere and a severe impairment of language production (Broca 1861), can be considered a foundational paper in human neuropsychology. The methodological debate on lesion–symptom mapping that this case prompted was to last until the present day (Catani and Mesulam 2008).

Research on the cognitive consequences of lesions of the right hemisphere began later (Brain 1941) and has been a source of equally controversial positions. Despite decades of research the lesional bases of neglect within the right hemisphere still remain controversial. It is likely that a substantial part of the controversy stems from the use of inadequate theories and methods of lesion–symptom mapping (Bartolomeo 2006, 2012).

7.1 Methodological Issues

The usual strategy for identifying the lesional correlates of neglect has been to use the lesion overlapping method. The technique is to superimpose the magnetic resonance or computed tomographic images of the lesions of a number of patients who had experienced a stroke and who either presented signs of neglect or not. The region of overlap of neglect patients is considered to be the essential lesional basis of this condition. To render the procedure more specific, one can also subtract from

P. Bartolomeo, *Attention Disorders After Right Brain Damage*,
DOI 10.1007/978-1-4471-5649-9_7, © Springer-Verlag London 2014

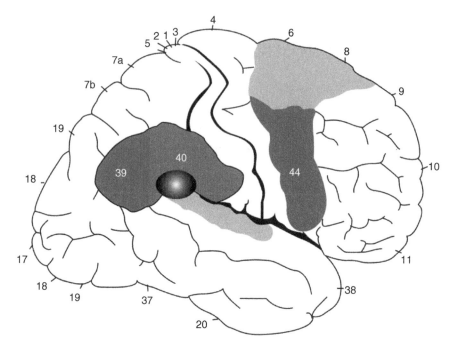

Fig. 7.1 Lesion localizations (*gray areas*) in stroke patients with left neglect according to classical lesion overlapping studies. In most patients, lesions overlap on the IPL (BA 39 and 40) and TPJ (*oval region* in the figure). In a minority of patients, neglect is consequent to damage to the dorsolateral and ventrolateral PFC. According to another study (Karnath et al. 2001), the critical zone of overlap is not parietal, but situated in the central sectors of the superior temporal gyrus (*light gray* region under the lateral sulcus) (Reproduced from Halligan et al. (2003). © 2003, with permission from Elsevier)

the overlap the lesions of patients free from neglect signs. These studies (Vallar and Perani 1986; Mort et al. 2003) have usually indicated the IPL and the TPJ as the sites of maximal lesion overlapping in the right hemisphere of the majority of patients (Fig. 7.1).

Contradictory evidence obtained with the same methods, however, pointed rather to a crucial role of lesions of the middle and rostral parts of the superior temporal gyrus and excluded a role for parietal lesions (Karnath et al. 2001). Nevertheless, damage to several other brain structures has been reported in cases of neglect, including the thalamus, the basal ganglia, and the dorsolateral PFC (Vallar 2001; Karnath et al. 2002).

In fact, consistent with the multifarious nature of their symptoms, patients with neglect often have relatively large lesions, which are likely to disrupt several functional modules. Indeed, regions in virtually the whole territory of the middle cerebral artery in the right hemisphere have been variously implicated in neglect signs in different studies (Fig. 7.2).

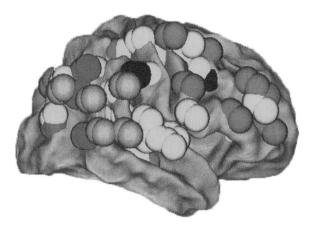

Fig. 7.2 Overview of all regions associated with unilateral spatial neglect, based upon 20 lesion mapping studies in the meta-analysis by Molenberghs et al. (2012). *Purple spheres* neglect tested with line bisection tasks, *red spheres* neglect tested with cancellation tasks, *green spheres* neglect tested with a combination of tasks, *blue spheres* allocentric neglect, *black spheres* personal neglect, *orange spheres* spatial extinction (Figure as originally published in Molenberghs et al. (2012))

The lesion overlap method used for human studies, with its emphasis on focal hot spots (Molenberghs et al. 2012), has several problems (Godefroy et al. 1998; Bartolomeo 2006, 2011). An obvious first limitation is the lack of spatial resolution, resulting from the coarse boundaries of vascular lesions. Poor spatial resolution is aggravated by the fact that lesions are usually plotted, or "normalized," on a standard brain, which can only approximate the spatial arrangement of real individual brains. Second, vascular lesions may well reflect differences in vascular territories rather than true functional organization of the brain. Third, in the case of multiple lesions, by no means a rare occurrence in neglect, the region of overlap may be identified as the crucial region, whereas the deficit may in fact result from the co-occurrence of distinct lesions. More generally, the voxel-based statistics used by the lesion overlapping method relies on the assumption that the voxels of maximum overlap correspond to the crucial cortical correlate of the neurological deficit. While this may well be the case, it is also possible, according to a perspective taking into proper account the network-based nature of most brain systems, that lesions located in different sites along the trajectory of a white matter pathway impair the integrated functioning of the cortical network connected by that pathway (Catani and Mesulam 2008). In this case, the lesion overlap method would be clearly inadequate to identify the brain network at issue (Bartolomeo 2006). Another critical variable, rarely mentioned in studies on stroke patients, is the time since stroke. Acute patients are more likely to suffer from diaschisis phenomena (Feeney and Baron 1986), with dysfunction of anatomically intact regions distant from the lesion but connected to it. Chronic patients' results, on the other hand, may be contaminated by compensation strategies (Bartolomeo 1997).

7.2 Voxel-Based Lesion–Symptom Mapping (VLSM)

Voxel-based lesion–symptom mapping (Bates et al. 2003), in comparison to the lesion overlap method, is a more quantitative method of structure–function correlation, inspired by functional neuroimaging studies. After brain normalization to a standard template, patients are classified into two groups according to which voxels are damaged. Neuropsychological scores are then compared between the two groups, yielding a statistical evaluation for each voxel (e.g., t-tests for continuous measures or Fisher tests for binary scores). Statistical results evaluating patients' performance on a voxel-by-voxel basis can then be drawn on brain maps with color codes indicating the probability that damage to that voxel has to produce the neuropsychological deficit. When applied to a group of 80 patients with right hemisphere stroke (Verdon et al. 2006), VLSM demonstrated that lateralized deficits of performance on different neglect tasks correlated with damage in different brain areas. For example, consistent with previous clinical-anatomical investigations (Binder et al. 1992), ipsilesional bias in line bisection was associated with posterior occipitoparietal lesions, whereas deficits in multiple-item cancellation were observed in patients with frontal damage. Importantly, however, damage to frontoparietal white matter fibers, which the authors identified with the pathway described by Thiebaut de Schotten et al. (2005) (see the following Sect. 7.3), correlated with the presence of generalized and severe neglect.

VLSM provides more quantitative and rigorous data than the lesion overlapping method, but the resulting maps suffer from many of the same shortcomings. In particular, the underlying theoretical assumptions are similar and based on a localist approach which considers brain functions as being associated to specific cortical regions rather than being network based (Catani and ffytche 2005).

7.3 Frontoparietal Networks

In short, the lesion overlapping and voxel-based approaches tend to rely on a localist view of anatomo-functional relationships, according to which each brain region is dedicated to, and crucial for, a particular function. Much evidence from cognitive neuroscience suggests, rather, that the brain is a mosaic of functionally distributed and highly interactive regions. As a consequence, the function of a given brain region may only emerge through the interaction with other regions, in a functional network organization. This is certainly true of the large-scale brain networks which subtend attentional processes (see Sect. 1.1). If this is so, the lesion overlapping and VLSM methods might not be conducive to accurate anatomo-clinical correlations (Bartolomeo 2011).

Recent studies have employed alternative methods to investigate the neural bases of neglect. Thiebaut de Schotten et al. (2005) combined diffusion tensor imaging (DTI) tractography, a technique which visualizes in vivo the white matter fiber tracts (Basser et al. 1994), with direct electrical stimulation of the brain (Duffau et al. 1999). When removing a brain tumor, the surgeon tries to perform a resection which is as radical as possible, without leaving the patient with a neurological deficit. To accomplish this, the patient is awakened during the intervention, and small brain regions (approximately 5 mm) are temporarily inactivated with electrical stimuli while the patient performs functional tasks. If the patient produces incorrect responses, the surgeon leaves the region intact, to preserve the patient's functional abilities.

Thiebaut de Schotten et al. (2005) asked two such patients to bisect 20-cm horizontal lines while being operated of a low-grade glioma in the right hemisphere. Patients deviated rightward upon inactivation of the supramarginal gyrus (the rostral subdivision of the IPL, see Fig. 1.2.) and of the caudal part of the superior temporal gyrus, but performed accurately when more rostral portions of the superior temporal gyrus or the FEF were inactivated. More importantly, however, the strongest deviations occurred in one patient upon inactivation of a white matter region in the depth of the IPL, after most of the tumor had been removed. To map the course of long association fibers in the white matter of this particular patient, DTI tractography was used in postoperative MRI images. The tract whose inactivation had brought about the maximal rightward deviation likely corresponded to the human homologous of the second branch of the SLF, or SLF II (see Sect. 1.1; Schmahmann and Pandya 2006; Thiebaut de Schotten et al. 2011). These findings on the importance of SLF damage in neglect were later confirmed by reanalyses of previous studies on stroke patients, where white matter damage was often present but overlooked (Bartolomeo et al. 2007; Thiebaut de Schotten et al. 2008) (Fig. 7.3).

This evidence confirmed and specified the previous results of Doricchi and Tomaiuolo (2003), who found a maximum lesion overlap on locations compatible with the trajectory of the SLF in stroke patients with neglect (see also Leibovitch et al. 1998), and was later replicated in other neurosurgical patients by Vallar et al. (2013).

Thus, several lines of evidence demonstrated an associated injury in white matter pathways connecting frontoparietal networks in monkey studies (Gaffan and Hornak 1997) and in human neglect patients with vascular damage (Urbanski et al. 2008, 2011; Chechlacz et al. 2010; Verdon et al. 2010; Thiebaut de Schotten et al. 2012) or neurosurgical lesions (Thiebaut de Schotten et al. 2005). It must be noted that in all the studies on human brain-damaged patients cited here, the lesions affected both the gray and the white matter. However, a recent single case report demonstrated that severe, if transitory, neglect signs can result from small lesions restricted to the white matter and affecting components of the SLF (Ciaraffa et al. 2013) (Fig. 7.4).

Altogether, this accumulated evidence suggests that neglect signs do not result from focal cortical lesions, but correlate with dysfunction of large-scale networks, whose nodes include the PPC, the lateral PFC, the TPJ, and the occipital lobe (Bartolomeo et al. 2007; Doricchi et al. 2008). As mentioned in Sect. 1.1, these cortical nodes show increased BOLD response during spatial orienting of attention (Nobre 2001; Corbetta and Shulman 2002; Bartolomeo et al. 2008) (Fig. 7.5).

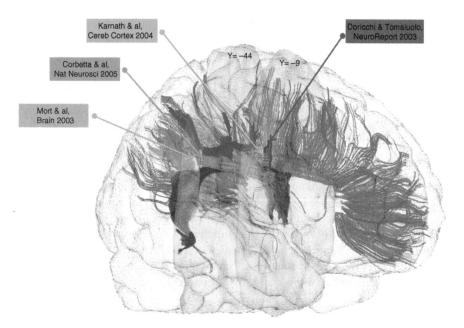

Fig. 7.3 The maximum (Karnath et al. 2004) overlap spots of lesion overlapping studies of neglect in stroke patients are plotted on the normal architecture of branches of the SLF and the corpus callosum, obtained through DTI tractography (Bartolomeo et al. 2007). In all the reported studies, lesion overlap occurred at or near the second branch (in *blue*) and the third branch (in *ochre*) of the SLF. *Red*, corpus callosum; *dark blue*, arcuate fasciculus (Reproduced from Bartolomeo et al. (2007). © 2007, with permission from Oxford University Press).

However, despite the obvious links between left neglect and dysfunction of large-scale frontoparietal networks in the right hemisphere (Bartolomeo 2006, 2007; Doricchi et al. 2008), the most severe and persistent signs of left neglect typically occur after retrorolandic lesions. This apparent paradox may depend on the architecture of frontoparietal connections in the human brain.

As mentioned in Sect. 1.1, the SLF II, whose caudal cortical origin is in part shared with that of the SLF III in the IPL, connects the parietal component of the VAN to the prefrontal component of the DAN (Thiebaut de Schotten et al. 2011) (see Fig. 7.5). Thus, it is plausible that damage to the IPL (Mort et al. 2003), when accompanied by injury to the underlying white matter (Doricchi and Tomaiuolo 2003; Verdon et al. 2010), can produce severe and persisting signs of neglect because it can jointly disrupt the functioning of the VAN (through SLF III disconnection) and of its communication with the DAN (through SLF II damage). On the other hand, less extensive lesions, perhaps sparing a significant part of SLF II, might allow for intra-hemispheric compensation mechanisms relying on the possibility of communication between VAN and DAN offered by SLF II. In this case, an initial imbalance between the dorsal frontoparietal networks, with the left hemisphere DAN being relatively more active than its right hemisphere counterpart, might subside after the acute phase with consequent recovery from neglect signs (Corbetta et al. 2005).

Fig. 7.4 Lesions (in *white*) confined to the white matter in the patient described by Ciaraffa et al. (2013). Virtual dissection with DTI-MR tractography showing the trajectories of the three segments of the bilateral arcuate fasciculus, right inferior frontal occipital fasciculus (IFOF), and right uncinate fasciculus projected over axial diffusion-weighted magnetic resonance images at the level of the midbrain (*top panel*), splenium of the corpus callosum (*middle panel*), and corona radiata (*bottom panel*). Note the relationship of the acute infarcts with the right arcuate fasciculus at multiple levels. Ischemic infarcts have involved the long and posterior segments (*top, middle*), the corona radiata, and the anterior segment of the arcuate fasciculus (*bottom*). Virtual dissection of the three segments of the arcuate fasciculus shows moderate asymmetry of the direct segments with the left-sided arcuate fasciculus being larger than the right-sided one. The fasciculi are color coded: arcuate fasciculus segments (long, *red*; anterior, *green*; posterior, *yellow*), IFOF (*orange*), and uncinate fasciculus (*cyan*) (Reproduced from Ciaraffa et al. (2013), http://www. tandfonline.com/doi/full/10.1 080/13554794.2012.667130. © 2013, with permission from Taylor & Francis Ltd)

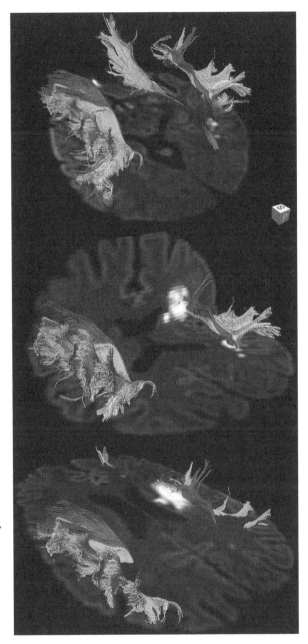

Thiebaut de Schotten et al. (2012) investigated the lesional antecedents of chronic neglect in 58 patients with strokes in the territory of the right middle cerebral artery. The results showed that the most sensitive and specific predictors of chronic persistence of neglect, which occurred in 38 patients, were damage to SLF

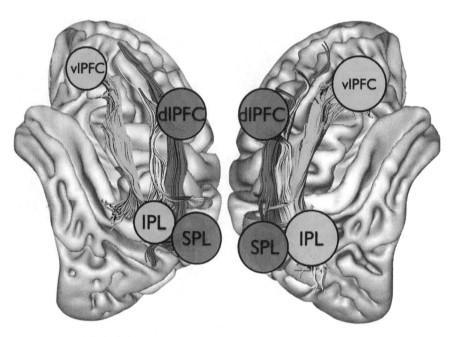

Fig. 7.5 Schematic depiction of frontoparietal attentional networks for visuospatial processing in the two hemispheres, based on Corbetta and Shulman (2002) and Thiebaut de Schotten et al. (2011). *IPL* and *SPL*, inferior and superior parietal lobules, *dlPFC* and *vlPFC* dorsolateral and ventrolateral prefrontal cortex. The size of the cortical nodes and of their connections symbolizes their putative importance in visuospatial processing (Figure as originally published in Bartolomeo et al. (2012))

II and (although less robustly) SLF III. Lesion size and the presence of visual field defects could not explain this result, because they were covaried out. Among the 38 patients with chronic neglect, only 7 did not have lesions consistent with frontoparietal SLF disconnection. All of these patients had a focal lesion in the lateral–dorsal portion of the thalamus, which connects the premotor cortex with the IPL. In the same study, the authors also performed a complete in vivo tractography dissection of white matter pathways in 2 further patients, 1 with and the other without signs of neglect. These two patients were studied both in the acute phase and one year after stroke and were perfectly matched for age, handedness, stroke onset, lesion size, and cortical lesion involvement. Importantly, only the patient with neglect had tractography signs of frontoparietal disconnection. Thus, this study strongly supported the hypothesis that anatomical disconnections leading to a functional breakdown of frontoparietal networks are an important pathophysiological factor leading to chronic left spatial neglect. Thiebaut de Schotten et al. (2012) also proposed that different loci of SLF disconnection on the rostrocaudal axis can be associated with disconnection of short-range white matter pathways within the frontal or parietal areas (Fig. 7.6). Such different local disconnection patterns can thus play a role in the important clinical variability among neglect patients.

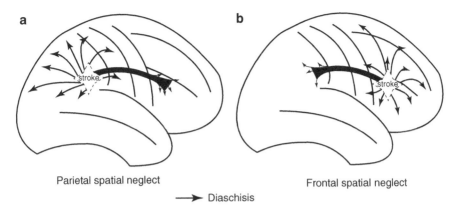

Fig. 7.6 A diaschetic model of neglect dissociations after parietal or frontal lesions, according to Thiebaut de Schotten et al. (2012). (**a**) Parietal and (**b**) frontal strokes interrupting long-range frontoparietal connections, and resulting in general hypoactivation of the frontoparietal attentional networks, can also interrupt short-range connections and thus determine local dysfunction of the neighboring areas in the parietal or in the frontal lobe, thus producing different patterns of performance in neglect patients (Reproduced from Thiebaut de Schotten et al. (2012). © 2012, with permission from Oxford University Press)

7.4   Callosal Neglect

As originally suggested by Norman Geschwind (1965), an isolated left hemisphere might in some cases take over the control of performance, with consequent rightward attentional bias (Berlucchi et al. 1997; Bartolomeo et al. 2007). Consistent with these notions, damage to the anterior portions of the corpus callosum (genu and trunk) may determine response-related left neglect for tasks performed with the right hand (Kashiwagi et al. 1990; Pouget et al. 2011). On the other hand, damage to the posterior callosal splenium, when occurring together with damage to the visual cortex or the visual pathways in the right hemisphere, may determine left neglect signs through a deafferentation, because such lesions would completely deprive the left hemisphere of visual information coming from the left visual field. This pattern has been documented both in monkeys (Gaffan and Hornak 1997) and in human patients (Park et al. 2006; Tomaiuolo et al. 2010). Although surgical section of the corpus callosum does not typically determine signs of neglect (Berlucchi et al. 1997; but see Corballis et al. 2005), it may do so in patients with previous right hemisphere damage (Heilman and Adams 2003). In the latter case, callosal disconnection presumably prevents the left hemisphere from compensating for the deficits induced by right hemisphere damage by taking charge of left-sided events (Bartolomeo et al. 2007). In agreement with these notions, microstructural damage of the posterior corpus callosum has been shown to correlate with the clinical severity of neglect as shown by patients' scores on a paper-and-pencil test battery (Bozzali et al. 2012).

7.5   More Ventral Networks

Less commonly, signs of neglect can result from damage in regions ventral to the frontoparietal networks described above. For example, signs of neglect can also result from a combined lesion of the visual pathways in one hemisphere and of the splenium of the corpus callosum. Gaffan and Hornak (1997) demonstrated that monkeys with combined resection of the right optic tract (causing complete left hemianopia) and of the corpus callosum (causing complete interhemispheric fore-brain disconnection) showed more severe neglect than monkeys undergoing section of frontoparietal connections (also determining substantial neglect) or resection of the parietal and/or prefrontal cortex (resulting in very mild and transitory neglect). The authors argued that severe neglect in monkeys with combined optic tract–callosal disconnection depended on the impossibility of the intact attentional fron-toparietal system of the blind hemisphere to receive the visual information gathered by the seeing hemisphere.

Park et al. (2006) reported on 45 patients with brain damage in the vascular ter-ritory of the right or left posterior cerebral artery, tested in the subacute phase (within 2 months of stroke). Signs of contralesional neglect were present in 48 % of the right brain-damaged patients and in 35 % of the patients with left hemisphere damage; however, the severity of neglect was greater in the right hemisphere group. Lesion analysis demonstrated that the association of right occipital injury with sple-nial damage was critical for the development of left neglect; occipital damage alone was only rarely associated with neglect. Tomaiuolo et al. (2010) described two patients with strokes in the territory of the posterior cerebral artery, which caused selective damage to the splenium of the corpus callosum and the adjacent right pri-mary visual cortex. Both patients had severe neglect restricted to the visual domain, without any evidence of personal, motor, or imaginal neglect.

As mentioned in Sect. 1.1.4, two major rostrocaudal white matter pathways run in the depth of the occipital and temporal lobes, the inferior longitudinal fasciculus (ILF) which connects the occipital and temporal poles, and the inferior fronto-occipital fasciculus (IFOF) which connects occipital regions with the ventrolateral PFC and the medial orbitofrontal cortex (Catani et al. 2003) (see Fig. 1.7).

A maximum lesion overlap on the white matter was also reported in the rel-atively rare cases of neglect resulting from lesions in the territory of the right posterior cerebral artery (Mort et al. 2003; Park et al. 2006). Bird et al. (2006) described overlap location as compatible with the trajectory of the ILF. Using DTI tractography, Urbanski et al. (2008) performed in vivo reconstruction of the SLF, the ILF, and the IFOF in four patients with right brain lesions. DTI evidence of IFOF disconnection was present only in the two patients showing signs of left neglect. This result was subsequently confirmed in a larger sample of 12 right brain-damaged patients, of whom six showed signs of left neglect (Urbanski et al. 2011). In this study, the IFOF was disconnected in all patients with neglect and was normal and symmetrical in all patients without neglect. It must be noted, how-ever, that some patients with IFOF disconnection do not show signs of neglect

(Thiebaut de Schotten et al. 2012). Thus, damage to the IFOF might not be necessary by itself to produce signs of neglect, but it might well contribute to neglect signs. Possible mechanisms of the contribution of IFOF damage to neglect could be a deprivation of visual cortex of top-down modulation from more anterior regions or a decrease of the influence of visual input on the right ventrolateral PFC, with consequent deterioration of patients' level of alertness (Urbanski et al. 2008).

7.6 Lesional Correlates of Specific Forms of Neglect

There have been several attempts to define the lesional correlates of specific forms of neglect. The results of these studies are not always consistent, perhaps because of the previously mentioned problems associated with the identification of lesional correlates of network-based deficits.

Thus, the already mentioned VLSM study of 80 patients by Verdon et al. (2010) found evidence suggesting a preferential involvement of the IPL for perceptive/visuospatial components of neglect (such as those associated with impaired text reading, line bisection, and drawing), of the dorsolateral PFC for an exploratory/visuomotor component (e.g., in target cancellation tasks), and of deep temporal lobe regions for the allocentric/object-based component (object-based neglect in the Ota cancellation task). Another VLSM study (Committeri et al. 2007) explored the personal/extrapersonal dichotomy and associated impaired processing of extrapersonal space with damage to the ventral premotor cortex, middle frontal gyrus, and superior temporal regions, whereas personal neglect resulted from lesion of inferior parietal regions (supramarginal gyrus, postcentral gyrus and especially the underlying white matter). Of note, the neglect test battery did not include line bisection. Hillis et al. (2005) studied 50 patients with hyperacute (within 48 h of onset) subcortical infarcts in the right hemisphere with diffusion-weighted and perfusion-weighted MRI. They used the test developed by Ota et al. (2001) and found that omissions in the left part of the sheet (scene-based neglect, see Sect. 5.2.3) were associated with hypoperfusion of the angular gyrus, whereas object-based neglect on the same task was associated with hypoperfusion of the superior temporal gyrus. By using a conceptually similar test with 41 chronic stage patients (>9 months post injury), Chechlacz et al. (2010) came to the partly different conclusion that object-based neglect was associated with damage to posterior cortical regions (posterior superior temporal sulcus, angular, middle temporal, and middle occipital gyri). In contrast, egocentric neglect was associated with more anterior cortical damage (middle frontal, postcentral, supramarginal, and superior temporal gyri) and damage to subcortical structures. There were regions, such as IPS and TPJ, whose damage was associated with both forms of neglect. Importantly, damage to long association and projection white matter pathways such as the SLF, ILF, IFOF, thalamic radiations, and corona radiata was also associated with generalized neglect.

The anatomy of imaginal neglect has not been thoroughly explored. Many cases have large right hemisphere lesions centered on the temporoparietal region, similar to those observed in patients with visuospatial neglect (Bisiach et al. 1981; Bartolomeo et al. 1994). Single patients with isolated imaginal neglect had lesions in the dorsolateral PFC (Guariglia et al. 1993) or in the thalamus (Ortigue et al. 2001). A case study of a patient with an association of imaginal and visuospatial neglect (Rode et al. 2010) found evidence consistent with the possibility that disconnection factors might also contribute to imaginal neglect. Diffusion MRI in this patient found evidence for intra-hemispheric connections in the SLF and in the IFOF, consistent with previous reports on patients with visuospatial neglect (see above Sects. 7.3 and 7.4). In addition, there was impaired microstructural integrity of the splenium of the callosum corpus. A control patient with visuospatial but not imaginal neglect had only intra-hemispheric disconnection. This evidence needs to be confirmed on a larger patient series, but it suggests that imaginal neglect may result from the concomitant presence of (1) frontoparietal dysfunction impairing orienting towards left-sided items and (2) posterior callosal disconnection preventing the symmetrical processing of spatial information from long-term memory. Indeed, TMS evidence in normal participants suggests that the two parietal lobes have different roles in spatial imagery (Sack et al. 2005). The left parietal lobe might be important during the early stages of generation of spatial images, whereas the right parietal lobe could later carry out spatial operations on these images. On the other hand, in brain-damaged patients splenial disconnection per se does not seem a sufficient condition for imaginal neglect to emerge, as shown by two patients with splenial disconnection and lesions of the visual pathways or of the visual cortex leading to hemianopia, who had signs of perceptual neglect but no imaginal neglect (Tomaiuolo et al. 2010).

References

Bartolomeo P. The novelty effect in recovered hemineglect. Cortex. 1997;33:323–32.
Bartolomeo P. A parieto-frontal network for spatial awareness in the right hemisphere of the human brain. Arch Neurol. 2006;63:1238–41.
Bartolomeo P. Visual neglect. Curr Opin Neurol. 2007;20:381–6.
Bartolomeo P. The quest for the 'critical lesion site' in cognitive deficits: problems and perspectives. Cortex. 2011;47:1010–2.
Bartolomeo P. The elusive nature of white matter damage in anatomo-clinical correlations. Front Hum Neurosci. 2012;6:229.
Bartolomeo P, D'Erme P, Gainotti G. The relationship between visuospatial and representational neglect. Neurology. 1994;44:1710–4.
Bartolomeo P, Thiebaut de Schotten M, Doricchi F. Left unilateral neglect as a disconnection syndrome. Cereb Cortex. 2007;45:3127–48.
Bartolomeo P, Zieren N, Vohn R, Dubois B, Sturm W. Neural correlates of primary and reflective consciousness of spatial orienting. Neuropsychologia. 2008;46:348–61.
Bartolomeo P, Thiebaut Schotten M, Chica AB. Brain networks of visuospatial attention and their disruption in visual neglect. Human. Neuroscience. 2012;6:110.
Basser PJ, Mattiello J, LeBihan D. MR diffusion tensor spectroscopy and imaging. Biophys J. 1994;66:259–67.

Bates E, Wilson SM, Saygin AP, Dick F, Sereno MI, Knight RT, Dronkers NF. Voxel-based lesion-symptom mapping. Nat Neurosci. 2003;6:448–50.

Berlucchi G, Aglioti S, Tassinari G. Rightward attentional bias and left hemisphere dominance in a cue-target light detection task in a callosotomy patient. Neuropsychologia. 1997;35:941–52.

Binder J, Marshall R, Lazar R, Benjamin J, Mohr JP. Distinct syndromes of hemineglect. Arch Neurol. 1992;49:1187–94.

Bird C, Malhotra P, Parton A, Coulthard EJ, Rushworth MF, Husain M. Visual neglect after right posterior cerebral artery infarction. J Neurol Neurosurg Psychiatry. 2006;77:1008–12.

Bisiach E, Capitani E, Luzzatti C, Perani D. Brain and conscious representation of outside reality. Neuropsychologia. 1981;19:543–51.

Bozzali M, Mastropasqua C, Cercignani M, Giulietti G, Bonni S, Caltagirone C, Koch G. Microstructural damage of the posterior corpus callosum contributes to the clinical severity of neglect. PLoS One. 2012;7:e48079.

Brain RW. Visual disorientation with special reference to lesion of the right brain hemisphere. Brain. 1941;64:244–72.

Broca PP. Perte de la parole, ramollissement chronique et destruction partielle du lobe antérieur gauche. Bulletin de la Société Anthropologique. 1861;2:235–8.

Catani M, ffytche DH. The rises and falls of disconnection syndromes. Brain. 2005;128:2224–39.

Catani M, Mesulam M-M. The arcuate fasciculus and the disconnection theme in language and aphasia: history and current state. Cortex. 2008;44:953–61.

Catani M, Jones DK, Donato R, Ffytche DH. Occipito-temporal connections in the human brain. Brain. 2003;126:2093–107.

Chechlacz M, Rotshtein P, Bickerton WL, Hansen PC, Deb S, Humphreys GW. Separating neural correlates of allocentric and egocentric neglect: distinct cortical sites and common white matter disconnections. Cogn Neuropsychol. 2010;27:277–303.

Ciaraffa F, Castelli G, Parati EA, Bartolomeo P, Bizzi A. Visual neglect as a disconnection syndrome? A confirmatory case report. Neurocase. 2013;19(4):351–9.

Committeri G, Pitzalis S, Galati G, Patria F, Pelle G, Sabatini U, Castriota-Scanderbeg A, Piccardi L, Guariglia C, Pizzamiglio L. Neural bases of personal and extrapersonal neglect in humans. Brain. 2007;130:431–41.

Corballis MC, Corballis PM, Fabri M, Paggi A, Manzoni T. Now you see it, now you don't: variable hemineglect in a commissurotomized man. Cogn Brain Res. 2005;25:521–30.

Corbetta M, Shulman GL. Control of goal-directed and stimulus-driven attention in the brain. Nat Rev Neurosci. 2002;3:201–15.

Corbetta M, Kincade MJ, Lewis C, Snyder AZ, Sapir A. Neural basis and recovery of spatial attention deficits in spatial neglect. Nat Neurosci. 2005;8:1603–10.

Doricchi F, Tomaiuolo F. The anatomy of neglect without hemianopia: a key role for parietal-frontal disconnection? NeuroReport. 2003;14:2239–43.

Doricchi F, Thiebaut de Schotten M, Tomaiuolo F, Bartolomeo P. White matter (dis)connections and gray matter (dys)functions in visual neglect: gaining insights into the brain networks of spatial awareness. Cortex. 2008;44:983–95.

Duffau H, Capelle L, Sichez J, Faillot T, Abdennour L, Law Koune JD, Dadoun S, Bitar A, Arthuis F, Van Effenterre R, Fohanno D. Intra-operative direct electrical stimulations of the central nervous system: the Salpêtrière experience with 60 patients. Acta Neurochir. 1999;141:1157–67.

Feeney DM, Baron JC. Diaschisis. Stroke. 1986;17:817–30.

Gaffan D, Hornak J. Visual neglect in the monkey. Representation and disconnection. Brain. 1997;120:1647–57.

Geschwind N. Disconnexion syndromes in animals and man – part I. Brain. 1965;88:237–94.

Godefroy O, Duhamel A, Leclerc X, Saint Michel T, Henon H, Leys D. Brain-behaviour relationships. Some models and related statistical procedures for the study of brain-damaged patients. Brain. 1998;121(Pt 8):1545–56.

Guariglia C, Padovani A, Pantano P, Pizzamiglio L. Unilateral neglect restricted to visual imagery. Nature. 1993;364:235–7.

Halligan PW, Fink GR, Marshall JC, Vallar G. Spatial cognition: evidence from visual neglect. Trends Cogn Sci. 2003;7:125–33.

Heilman KM, Adams DJ. Callosal neglect. Arch Neurol. 2003;60:276–9.

Hillis AE, Newhart M, Heidler J, Barker PB, Herskovits EH, Degaonkar M. Anatomy of spatial attention: insights from perfusion imaging and hemispatial neglect in acute stroke. J Neurosci. 2005;25:3161–7.

Karnath H-O, Ferber S, Himmelbach M. Spatial awareness is a function of the temporal not the posterior parietal lobe. Nature. 2001;411:950–63.

Karnath H-O, Himmelbach M, Rorden C. The subcortical anatomy of human spatial neglect: putamen, caudate nucleus and pulvinar. Brain. 2002;125:350–60.

Karnath H-O, Fruhmann Berger M, Kuker W, Rorden C. The anatomy of spatial neglect based on voxelwise statistical analysis: a study of 140 patients. Cerebral Cortex. 2004;14:1164–72.

Kashiwagi A, Kashiwagi T, Nishikawa T, Tanabe H, Okuda J. Hemispatial neglect in a patient with callosal infarction. Brain. 1990;113:1005–23.

Leibovitch FS, Black SE, Caldwell CB, Ebert PL, Ehrlich LE, Szalai JP. Brain-behavior correlations in hemispatial neglect using CT and SPECT: the Sunnybrook Stroke Study. Neurology. 1998;50:901–8.

Molenberghs P, Sale MV, Mattingley JB. Is there a critical lesion site for unilateral spatial neglect? A meta-analysis using activation likelihood estimation. Front Hum Neurosci. 2012;6:78.

Mort DJ, Malhotra P, Mannan SK, Rorden C, Pambakian A, Kennard C, Husain M. The anatomy of visual neglect. Brain. 2003;126:1986–97.

Nobre AC. The attentive homunculus: now you see it, now you don't. Neurosci Biobehav Rev. 2001;25:477–96.

Ortigue S, Viaud-Delmon I, Annoni JM, Landis T, Michel C, Blanke O, Vuilleumier P, Mayer E. Pure representational neglect after right thalamic lesion. Ann Neurol. 2001;50:401–4.

Ota H, Fujii T, Suzuki K, Fukatsu R, Yamadori A. Dissociation of body-centered and stimulus-centered representations in unilateral neglect. Neurology. 2001;57:2064–9.

Park KC, Lee BH, Kim EJ, Shin MH, Choi KM, Yoon SS, Kwon SU, Chung CS, Lee KH, Heilman KM, Na DL. Deafferentation-disconnection neglect induced by posterior cerebral artery infarction. Neurology. 2006;66:56–61.

Pouget P, Pradat-Diehl P, Rivaud-Pechoux S, Wattiez N, Gaymard B. An oculomotor and computational study of a patient with diagonistic dyspraxia. Cortex. 2011;47:473–83.

Rode G, Cotton F, Revol P, Jacquin-Courtois S, Rossetti Y, Bartolomeo P. Representation and disconnection in imaginal neglect. Neuropsychologia. 2010;48:2903–11.

Sack AT, Camprodon JA, Pascual-Leone A, Goebel R. The dynamics of interhemispheric compensatory processes in mental imagery. Science. 2005;308:702–4.

Schmahmann JD, Pandya DN. Fiber pathways of the brain. New York: Oxford University Press; 2006.

Thiebaut de Schotten M, Tomaiuolo F, Aiello M, Merola S, Silvetti M, Lecce F, Bartolomeo P, Doricchi F. Damage to white matter pathways in sub-acute and chronic spatial neglect: a group study and two single-case studies with complete virtual "in-vivo" tractography dissection. Cereb Cortex. 2012.

Thiebaut de Schotten M, Urbanski M, Duffau H, Volle E, Levy R, Dubois B, Bartolomeo P. Direct evidence for a parietal-frontal pathway subserving spatial awareness in humans. Science. 2005;309:2226–8.

Thiebaut de Schotten M, Kinkingnéhun SR, Delmaire C, Lehéricy S, Duffau H, Thivard L, Volle E, Lévy R, Dubois B, Bartolomeo P. Visualization of disconnection syndromes in humans. Cortex. 2008;44:1097–103.

Thiebaut de Schotten M, Dell'Acqua F, Forkel SJ, Simmons A, Vergani F, Murphy DGM, Catani M. A lateralized brain network for visuospatial attention. Nat Neurosci. 2011;14:1245–6.

Tomaiuolo F, Voci L, Bresci M, Cozza S, Posteraro F, Oliva M, Doricchi F. Selective visual neglect in right brain damaged patients with splenial interhemispheric disconnection. Exp Brain Res. 2010;206:209–17.

Urbanski M, Thiebaut de Schotten M, Rodrigo S, Catani M, Oppenheim C, Touzé E, Chokron S, Méder J-F, Lévy R, Dubois B, Bartolomeo P. Brain networks of spatial awareness: evidence from diffusion tensor imaging tractography. J Neurol Neurosurg Psychiatry. 2008;79:598–601.

Urbanski M, Thiebaut de Schotten M, Rodrigo S, Oppenheim C, Touzé E, Méder JF, Moreau K, Loeper-Jeny C, Dubois B, Bartolomeo P. DTI-MR tractography of white matter damage in stroke patients with neglect. Exp Brain Res. 2011;208:491–505.

Vallar G. Extrapersonal visual unilateral spatial neglect and its neuroanatomy. Neuroimage. 2001;14:S52–8.

Vallar G, Perani D. The anatomy of unilateral neglect after right-hemisphere stroke lesions. A clinical/CT-scan correlation study in man. Neuropsychologia. 1986;24:609–22.

Vallar G, Bello L, Bricolo E, Castellano A, Casarotti A, Falini A, Riva M, Fava E, Papagno C. Cerebral correlates of visuospatial neglect: a direct cerebral stimulation study. Hum Brain Mapp. 2013.

Verdon V, Lovblad K-O, Hauert C-A, Vuilleumier P. Neuroanatomical basis of hemispatial neglect components using voxel-based lesion symptom mapping. In: 2nd meeting of the European Societies of Neuropsychology. Toulouse; 2006. p. 277.

Verdon V, Schwartz S, Lovblad KO, Hauert CA, Vuilleumier P. Neuroanatomy of hemispatial neglect and its functional components: a study using voxel-based lesion-symptom mapping. Brain. 2010;133:880–94.

Further Reading

Corbetta M, Shulman GL. Spatial neglect and attention networks. Annu Rev Neurosci. 2011;34: 569–99.

Doricchi F, Thiebaut de Schotten M, Tomaiuolo F, Bartolomeo P. White matter (dis)connections and gray matter (dys)functions in visual neglect: Gaining insights into the brain networks of spatial awareness. Cortex. 2008;44(8):983–95.

Molenberghs P, Sale MV, Mattingley JB. Is there a critical lesion site for unilateral spatial neglect? A meta-analysis using activation likelihood estimation. Front Hum Neurosci. 2012;6:78.

Chapter 8
Attention Disorders in Neurodegenerative Conditions

Keywords Alzheimer's disease • Corticobasal syndrome • Posterior cortical atrophy • Parkinsonian syndromes • Frontotemporal dementia

8.1 Clinical and Neuroscientific Relevance

The health systems of developed countries need to prepare for a general trend towards an increasingly aging population. It is estimated that by 2050, 106.2 million persons worldwide, or 1 in 85, will be living with Alzheimer's disease (AD) (Brookmeyer et al. 2007). The mainstream clinical diagnosis of AD continues to be mainly based on clinical criteria, although neuroimaging is beginning to be considered in new diagnostic algorithms (Dubois et al. 2007). The neuropsychological profile of AD characteristically includes early episodic memory loss, with accompanying neuroimaging evidence of medial temporal lobe atrophy. Nevertheless, it is increasingly being recognized that other progressive neurodegenerative conditions, such as posterior cerebral atrophy (PCA), often share the typical pathological findings of AD, consisting of amyloid plaques and neurofibrillary tangles. However, in this condition the distribution of pathological changes is atypical compared to that of classic AD, with a preponderance of neurofibrillary tangles and senile plaques in occipital, parietal, and middle/inferior temporal cortices in PCA. This suggests that some PCA cases might constitute variant forms of AD with an atypical neocortical focal onset (von Gunten et al. 2006; Alladi et al. 2007).

Attention disorders are often present in these conditions and can substantially contribute to the clinical picture (Bartolomeo and Migliaccio in press). Thus, there are essential clinical implications, both for the diagnosis of patients and for a better assessment of the rationale backing the use of emerging or future treatments that might slow down disease progression. The study of these neurodegenerative syndromes is also important for the development of neurocognitive modelling. Traditionally, lesion–symptom mapping in neuropsychology has focused on the study of patients with focal vascular strokes (see Chap. 7). The study of

P. Bartolomeo, *Attention Disorders After Right Brain Damage*,
DOI 10.1007/978-1-4471-5649-9_8, © Springer-Verlag London 2014

neurodegenerative conditions offers an important complementary perspective (Bartolomeo 2011). As mentioned in Sect. 7.1, lesion location in stroke might reflect differences in vascular territories rather than true functional organization of the brain, which may lead to incorrect conclusions when associating anatomical areas with brain functions. The progression of neurodegenerative diseases, in contrast, appears to follow functionally linked systems along large-scale brain networks. Distinct anatomo-functional networks may be the target of particular disease forms (Seeley et al. 2009).

Elderly people sometimes complain of "loss of efficiency," which might be related to problems in visuospatial attention. Forgetting where objects are placed, having the impression of being unsafe while driving, and experiencing difficulties when in new places or navigating new routes are examples of attention problems which may occur during normal aging. In several neurodegenerative conditions, such as corticobasal syndrome (CBS), AD, and parkinsonian syndromes, visuospatial deficits can appear as part of a more complex cognitive impairment profile. In others, such as in PCA, they constitute the central core of the syndrome (Possin 2010; Migliaccio et al. 2012a; Bartolomeo and Migliaccio in press).

In typical amnesic AD, attention disorders can occur early along with memory deficits. Later in the course of the disease, signs of visual neglect may appear (Bartolomeo et al. 1998; Venneri et al. 1998). In some cases, attention disorders can even precede the typical amnesic syndrome (D'Erme et al. 1991(abstract)), especially in the early onset AD variant, which occurs before the age of 65 (Frisoni et al. 2007). More specifically, visuospatial attention deficits can have a central role in the impairment of higher-level cognitive processes involving visual and spatial memory. Patients with CBS can also show signs of visuospatial neglect (Silveri et al. 2011).

8.2 Occipitotemporal and Frontoparietal Systems in Degenerative Diseases

Visuospatial deficits in neurodegenerative conditions often develop and progress along the main dorsal or ventral cortical visual streams described in Sect. 1.1.4 (Migliaccio et al. 2012b). As mentioned, the distribution of neuropathology in neurodegeneration seems to follow specific trajectories for each syndrome, targeting specific cerebral networks (Seeley et al. 2009). Within this framework, the anatomical definition of ventral and dorsal variants can assist the clinician in making a correct "topographical" diagnosis (Migliaccio et al. 2012b). Given the correspondences between disease, anatomically damaged patterns and related cognitive impairment, the interpretation of neuropsychological tests of visuospatial cognition has important implications for differential diagnosis and for monitoring disease progression (Bartolomeo and Migliaccio in press).

For example, among the patients reported by Migliaccio et al. (2012b), a 62-year-old woman had been experiencing isolated difficulties in reading and writing for about 7 years. At the time of the study, she complained of episodes of topographical disorientation, and her neuropsychological profile was dominated by a severe visual impairment. She was unable to copy the Rey–Osterrieth figure and was impaired in face recognition tests. She performed poorly on reading words and pseudo-words. Despite her marked visual and gnosic difficulties, she had excellent episodic memory for recent events and no difficulty in remembering appointments. She had normal verbal working memory and oral language. The tractography study of this patient demonstrated white matter damage along all the main components of the ventral cortical visual stream (see Fig. 1.7), i.e., the ILF and the IFOF.

Another patient, a 58-year-old, right-handed medical doctor, was studied by Migliaccio et al. (2012a). Disease onset was characterized by multiple minor car accidents against left-sided obstacles, which would appear to suggest visual neglect as an early impairment. Clinical and neuropsychological examination 1.5 years after onset revealed signs of severe left visual neglect, along with optic ataxia and ocular apraxia, as well as left ideomotor apraxia. There was a 19 % rightward deviation on line bisection; performance was pathological on the landscape drawing copy and on the clock drawing test. There were rare left tactile extinctions on double stimulation. Mild memory impairment, especially with visuospatial material, and a very mild simultanagnosia were also present. Executive functions and calculation were relatively spared. MRI demonstrated bilateral cortical atrophy mainly located in the parietal lobes. In agreement with current clinical criteria (see Migliaccio et al. 2009), a diagnosis of PCA was made. During a 2-year follow-up, the neuropsychological profile remained highly asymmetric, with language and verbal memory largely preserved, while left visual neglect continued to represent the most severe symptom and remained a substantial source of handicap in her everyday life. DTI tractography of long-range white matter fibers demonstrated white matter damage largely restricted to the right hemisphere, including the SLF and the IFOF, whereas the homologous left-hemisphere tracts were spared (Fig. 8.1). The sparing of all the explored fasciculi in the left hemisphere, despite the cortical involvement of the occipital and parietal lobes, was consistent with the patient's cognitive profile, with relatively intact language and calculation abilities.

8.3   Spatial Attention in Degenerative Diseases

Visual neglect is especially frequent after focal vascular lesions of the right hemisphere (Chap. 7), but signs of neglect have been described in AD (Mendez et al. 1997; Bartolomeo et al. 1998; Venneri et al. 1998; Ishiai et al. 2000), CBS, and PCA. Out of 24 PCA patients, signs of neglect on at least one paper-and-pencil test were present in 16 patients, and 14 also had visual extinction or hemianopia (Andrade et al. 2010). Consistent with lesion–symptom mapping in patients with strokes in the territory of the right middle cerebral artery (Sect. 7.3), in PCA patients with left neglect, MRI-based DTI tractography demonstrated damage to frontoparietal white matter bundles in the right hemisphere (Migliaccio et al. 2012a, b) (see Fig. 8.1).

Inferior fronto-occipital fasciculus

Inferior longitudinal fasciculus

Superior longitudinal fasciculus

Corpus callosum

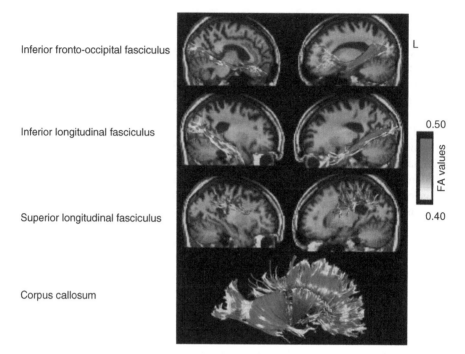

Fig. 8.1 Tractography study of the patient with PCA and left neglect reported by Migliaccio et al. (2012a). White matter tracts are rendered as maps of fractional anisotropy (*FA*, an index of microstructural white matter integrity) displayed on the native T1-weighted MRI for both hemispheres. FA values range from 0.40 (*yellow*, greater damage) to 0.50 (*red*, lesser damage). Damage was found in the right frontoparietal SLF. ILF and IFOF were also affected in the right hemisphere. There was also fiber loss in the posterior part of the corpus callosum (bottom panel, left side)". Left hemisphere tracts did not differ from age-matched controls (Reproduced from Migliaccio et al. (2012a). © 2012, with permission from Elsevier)

Among the variety of tests used in clinical practice (detailed in Chap. 4), line bisection might be more apt than other tests such as target cancellation to demonstrate neglect in patients with neurodegenerative conditions, such as PCA (Andrade et al. 2010), because performance on isolated horizontal lines is less prone to be influenced by other concomitant deficits such as simultanagnosia. In comparison with controls, PCA patients with signs of left-sided and right-sided neglect presented prominent hypoperfusion in right and left frontoparietal cortical networks, respectively (Andrade et al. 2012). In another study, on PCA patients rightward bias on the line bisection test was strongly correlated with atrophy and hypoperfusion in a large-scale frontoparietal network in the right hemisphere, involving the parieto-temporal cortex, the middle frontal gyrus, and in the postcentral region (Fig. 8.2) (Andrade et al. 2012). Thus, in these studies once again signs of neglect seemed to correlate with dysfunction in large-scale frontoparietal networks, beyond the sites of parietal atrophy (see also Migliaccio et al. 2012a, b), consistent with evidence from patients with vascular lesions (see above Sect. 7.3).

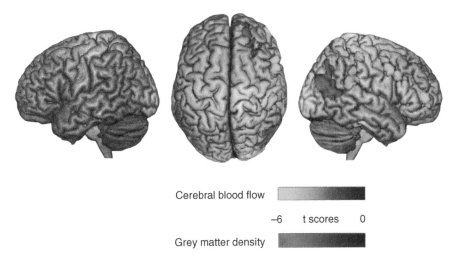

Cerebral blood flow

−6   t scores   0

Grey matter density

Fig. 8.2 Statistic parametric mapping results for 15 patients with PCA, who underwent brain MRI and SPECT and were required to bisect 20-cm long horizontal lines (Andrade et al. 2012). The figure displays the correlations between rightward deviations on line bisection, gray matter atrophy (in *red*), and regional brain hypoperfusion (*green*). These results indicate that, signs of left neglect in PCA are likely to depend on dysfunction of a large frontoparietal network in the right hemisphere, related to both cortical atrophy and decreased cerebral perfusion (Reproduced from Andrade et al. (2012). © 2012 with permission from BMJ Publishing Group Ltd)

The relative frequency of left- and right-sided neglect in neurodegenerative conditions is currently unknown. In some studies right-sided neglect was observed with an unexpected, relatively high frequency in neurodegenerative diseases as compared to its rarity in vascular patients (Bartolomeo et al. 1998; Andrade et al. 2010). Such a finding is in line with the proposal that damage to both hemispheres is more likely to cause signs of right-sided neglect than would unilateral damage of the left hemisphere (Weintraub et al. 1996). This might depend on damage to the right frontoparietal networks determining nonlateralized deficits, such as deficits of vigilant attention (see Sect. 1.2) which may be crucial for observing neglect signs (Husain and Nachev 2007). However, another study (Silveri et al. 2011) found that the usual predominance of left-sided neglect also occurred in degenerative patients.

Although visual extinction usually occurs after vascular strokes in the territory of medial cerebral artery (see Sect. 2.2), it has also been observed in neurodegenerative conditions such as PCA (Andrade et al. 2010). Also in neurodegenerative conditions the clinician must consider the possibility of normal performance on paper-and-pencil tests, despite the presence of more subtle disorder of visuospatial attention (Sect. 4.3). Such subclinical deficits of spatial attention (e.g., in RT performance) have been described in patients with AD (Parasuraman et al. 1992; Danckert et al. 1998; Balota and Faust 2001), Parkinson's disease (Wright et al. 1990; Cristinzio et al. 2013), Huntington's disease (Couette et al. 2008; Georgiou-Karistianis et al. 2012), and progressive supranuclear palsy (Rafal et al. 1988).

8.4   Control and Monitoring Deficits

Control and monitoring functions are mediated by cortical and subcortical frontal structures and by their connections with parietotemporal regions (see Sect. 1.3). Among neurodegenerative diseases, both AD and the frontal/behavioral variant of frontotemporal dementia (FTD) can especially impair these attention processes. Based on different patterns of neurodegeneration, particular clinical and cognitive profiles have been described in AD and FTD. Early memory impairment and subsequent language, praxic, and visuospatial deficits are typically present in AD.

In AD, the trajectory of damage includes the hippocampal and perihippocampal regions, where neurodegeneration originates with concomitant impairment of episodic memory, to the more posterior associative temporoparietal areas. Conversely, early changes in social conduct, insight, affective behavior, along with impaired initiative, verbal fluency, attention, planning, set shifting, problem solving, and working memory depend on pathological changes in the orbitofrontal and dorsolateral PFC, characteristically affected in patients with FTD (Rosen et al. 2002). Notwithstanding their profound biological, anatomical, and cognitive differences, AD and FTD seem to have similar consequences in executive functioning. Executive deficits reflect an impaired integration of the frontal lobes with different brain areas and in particular with more posterior brain regions. These functional and anatomical connections are damaged in both AD and FTD, thus perhaps accounting for their similarity in this specific domain. For this reason it might prove difficult to differentiate, on the basis of these functions, patients with FTD and AD, particularly when AD patients are younger and atypical (Bartolomeo and Migliaccio in press).

From the functional point of view, several large-scale brain networks, described as being dysfunctional in AD and FTD, are implicated in attention and monitoring behavior. These include networks implicated in salience processing (Seeley et al. 2007), executive processes (Seeley et al. 2008), attention/working memory processes (Damoiseaux et al. 2006), as well as the dorsal attention network (Fox et al. 2006). These networks are especially dysfunctional in FTD (Filippi et al. 2013). Impaired functioning of attention and monitoring networks may thus represent a pathophysiological signature of this disease.

Little is known about the potential occurrence of visuospatial attention deficits in FTD, although patients with vascular strokes in the frontal lobes can sometimes demonstrate signs of spatial neglect (Chap. 7). Note, however, that frontal damage in neglect typically implicates lateral frontal regions (see Figs. 7.1 and 7.2), i.e., the prefrontal nodes of the attention networks (see Figs. 1.3 and 7.5), whereas in the behavioral variant of FTD, the atrophy affects first and foremost the frontomedian brain regions, as well as the anterior insula and the thalamus (Schroeter et al. 2008). As a consequence, signs of visual neglect might not be as prominent in FTD as they are in PCA.

References

Alladi S, Xuereb J, Bak T, Nestor P, Knibb J, Patterson K, Hodges JR. Focal cortical presentations of Alzheimer's disease. Brain. 2007;130:2636–45.

Andrade K, Samri D, Sarazin M, Cruz De Souza L, Cohen L, Thiebaut de Schotten M, Dubois B, Bartolomeo P. Visual neglect in posterior cortical atrophy. BMC Neurol. 2010;10:68.

Andrade K, Kas A, Valabrègue R, Samri D, Sarazin M, Habert MO, Dubois B, Bartolomeo P. Visuospatial deficits in posterior cortical atrophy: structural and functional correlates. J Neurol Neurosurg Psychiatry. 2012;83:860–3.

Balota DA, Faust ME. Attention in dementia of the Alzheimer's type. In: Boller F, Grafman J, editors. Handbook of neuropsychology. 2nd ed. Amsterdam: Elsevier Science Publishers; 2001. p. 51–80.

Bartolomeo P. The quest for the 'critical lesion site' in cognitive deficits: problems and perspectives. Cortex. 2011;47:1010–2.

Bartolomeo P, Dalla Barba G, Boissé MT, Bachoud-Lévi AC, Degos JD, Boller F. Right-side neglect in Alzheimer's disease. Neurology. 1998;51:1207–9.

Bartolomeo P, Migliaccio R. Disorders of attentional processes. In: Husain M, Schott J, editors. Oxford textbook of cognitive neurology and dementia. Oxford: Oxford University Press (in press).

Brookmeyer R, Johnson E, Ziegler-Graham K, Arrighi HM. Forecasting the global burden of Alzheimer's disease. Alzheimers Dement. 2007;3:186–91.

Couette M, Bachoud-Lévi AC, Brugières P, Siéroff E, Bartolomeo P. Orienting of spatial attention in Huntington's disease. Neuropsychologia. 2008;46:1391–400.

Cristinzio C, Bononi M, Piacentini S, Albanese A, Bartolomeo P. Attentional networks in Parkinson's disease. Behavioural Neurology. 2013;27(4):495–500.

D'Erme P, Bartolomeo P, Masullo C. Alzheimer's disease presenting with visuo-spatial disorders. Ital J Neurol Sci. 1991 (abstract);12:117.

Damoiseaux JS, Rombouts SA, Barkhof F, Scheltens P, Stam CJ, Smith SM, Beckmann CF. Consistent resting-state networks across healthy subjects. Proc Natl Acad Sci U S A. 2006;103: 13848–53.

Danckert J, Maruff P, Crowe S, Currie J. Inhibitory processes in covert orienting in patients with Alzheimer's disease. Neuropsychology. 1998;12:225–41.

Dubois B, Feldman HH, Jacova C, Dekosky ST, Barberger-Gateau P, Cummings J, Delacourte A, Galasko D, Gauthier S, Jicha G, Meguro K, O'Brien J, Pasquier F, Robert P, Rossor M, Salloway S, Stern Y, Visser PJ, Scheltens P. Research criteria for the diagnosis of Alzheimer's disease: revising the NINCDS-ADRDA criteria. Lancet Neurol. 2007;6:734–46.

Filippi M, Agosta F, Scola E, Canu E, Magnani G, Marcone A, Valsasina P, Caso F, Copetti M, Comi G, Cappa SF, Falini A. Functional network connectivity in the behavioral variant of frontotemporal dementia. Cortex. 2013;49(9):2389–401.

Fox MD, Corbetta M, Snyder AZ, Vincent JL, Raichle ME. Spontaneous neuronal activity distinguishes human dorsal and ventral attention systems. Proc Natl Acad Sci U S A. 2006;103:10046–51.

Frisoni GB, Pievani M, Testa C, Sabattoli F, Bresciani L, Bonetti M, Beltramello A, Hayashi KM, Toga AW, Thompson PM. The topography of grey matter involvement in early and late onset Alzheimer's disease. Brain. 2007;130:720–30.

Georgiou-Karistianis N, Farrow M, Wilson-Ching M, Churchyard A, Bradshaw JL, Sheppard DM. Deficits in selective attention in symptomatic Huntington disease: assessment using an attentional blink paradigm. Cogn Behav Neurol. 2012;25:1–6.

Husain M, Nachev P. Space and the parietal cortex. Trends Cogn Sci. 2007;11:30–66.

Ishiai S, Koyama Y, Seki K, Orimo S, Sodeyama N, Ozawa E, Lee EY, Takahashi M, Watabiki S, Okiyama R, Ohtake T, Hiroki M. Unilateral spatial neglect in AD: significance of line bisection performance. Neurology. 2000;55:364–70.

Mendez MF, Cherrier MM, Cymerman JS. Hemispatial neglect on visual search tasks in Alzheimer's disease. Neuropsychiatry Neuropsychol Behav Neurol. 1997;10:203–8.

Migliaccio R, Agosta F, Rascovsky K, Karydas A, Bonasera S, Rabinovici GD, Miller BL, Gorno-Tempini ML. Clinical syndromes associated with posterior atrophy: early age at onset AD spectrum. Neurology. 2009;73:1571–8.

Migliaccio R, Agosta F, Toba MN, Samri D, Corlier F, de Souza LC, Chupin M, Sharman M, Gorno-Tempini ML, Dubois B, Filippi M, Bartolomeo P. Brain networks in posterior cortical atrophy: a single case tractography study and literature review. Cortex. 2012a;48:1298–309.

Migliaccio R, Agosta F, Scola E, Magnani G, Cappa SF, Pagani E, Canu E, Comi G, Falini A, Gorno-Tempini ML, Bartolomeo P, Filippi M. Ventral and dorsal visual streams in posterior cortical atrophy: a DT MRI study. Neurobiol Aging. 2012b;33:2572–84.

Parasuraman R, Greenwood PM, Haxby JV, Grady CL. Visuospatial attention dementia of the Alzheimer type. Brain. 1992;115(Pt 3):711–33.

Possin KL. Visual spatial cognition in neurodegenerative disease. Neurocase. 2010;16:466–87.

Rafal RD, Posner MI, Friedman JH, Inhoff AW, Bernstein E. Orienting of visual attention in progressive supranuclear palsy. Brain. 1988;111:267–80.

Rosen HJ, Gorno-Tempini ML, Goldman WP, Perry RJ, Schuff N, Weiner M, Feiwell R, Kramer JH, Miller BL. Patterns of brain atrophy in frontotemporal dementia and semantic dementia. Neurology. 2002;58:198–208.

Schroeter ML, Raczka K, Neumann J, von Cramon DY. Neural networks in frontotemporal dementia – a meta-analysis. Neurobiol Aging. 2008;29:418–26.

Seeley WW, Menon V, Schatzberg AF, Keller J, Glover GH, Kenna H, Reiss AL, Greicius MD. Dissociable intrinsic connectivity networks for salience processing and executive control. J Neurosci. 2007;27:2349–56.

Seeley WW, Crawford R, Rascovsky K, Kramer JH, Weiner M, Miller BL, Gorno-Tempini ML. Frontal paralimbic network atrophy in very mild behavioral variant frontotemporal dementia. Arch Neurol. 2008;65:249–55.

Seeley WW, Crawford RK, Zhou J, Miller BL, Greicius MD. Neurodegenerative diseases target large-scale human brain networks. Neuron. 2009;62:42–52.

Silveri MC, Ciccarelli N, Cappa A. Unilateral spatial neglect in degenerative brain pathology. Neuropsychology. 2011;25:554–66.

Venneri A, Pentore R, Cotticelli B, Della Sala S. Unilateral spatial neglect in the late stage of Alzheimer's disease. Cortex. 1998;34:743–52.

von Gunten A, Bouras C, Kovari E, Giannakopoulos P, Hof PR. Neural substrates of cognitive and behavioral deficits in atypical Alzheimer's disease. Brain Res Rev. 2006;51:176–211.

Weintraub S, Daffner KR, Ahern GL, Price BH, Mesulam MM. Right sided hemispatial neglect and bilateral cerebral lesions. J Neurol Neurosurg Psychiatry. 1996;60:342–4.

Wright MJ, Burns RJ, Geffen GM, Geffen LB. Covert orientation of visual attention in Parkinson's disease: an impairment in the maintenance of attention. Neuropsychologia. 1990;28:151–9.

Further Reading

Balota DA, Faust ME. Attention in dementia of the Alzheimer's type. In: Boller F, Grafman J, editors. Handbook of neuropsychology. 2nd ed. Amsterdam: Elsevier Science Publishers; 2001. p. 51–80.

Seeley WW, Crawford RK, Zhou J, Miller BL, Greicius MD. Neurodegenerative diseases target large-scale human brain networks. Neuron. 2009;62(1):42–52.

Chapter 9
Treatment of Attention Disorders

Keywords Scanning training • Vestibular stimulation • Alertness training • Prism adaptation • TMS • Noradrenergic agents • Dopaminergic agents • Anticholinesterasic agents

Despite the possibility for some patients with right hemisphere damage to compensate for their deficits, in others attention disorders assume a chronic character, with consequent substantial disability. Thus, in the past decades many forms of interventions have been proposed to remediate neglect, which is the most clinically relevant condition associated with right hemisphere damage, as well as a well-recognized predictor of poor functional outcome (Luaute et al. 2006a) (Fig. 9.1). In addition, numerous studies have shown how certain experimental stimulations could produce a transient remission of neglect signs (Chokron et al. 2007). Since some of these techniques have been used successfully in clinical practice, they will also be discussed here. As seen in Chap. 7, neglect signs do not result from focal cortical lesions, but from a more diffuse dysfunction of large-scale brain networks including not only the lesion but also anatomically intact nodes. The network-based nature of the lesions producing neglect opens the possibility to restore or rebalance network activity within and across the hemispheres by acting on the intact nodes of the damaged networks or on their left hemisphere homologues (Halligan and Bartolomeo 2012).

9.1 Top-Down Techniques

These techniques aim at stimulating top-down exploration processes of visual scanning, so that patients pay attention to the neglected side (e.g., looking at a left-sided red bar before reading a text). These techniques obviously require some degree of awareness of disease on the patient's part, which is not always present because of anosognosia. Moreover, if these techniques can improve the level of awareness of

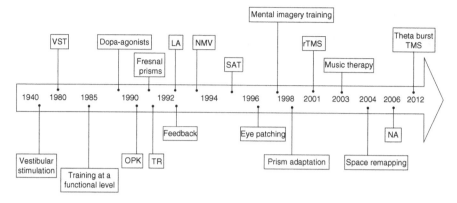

Fig. 9.1 Timeline of the first publications for different attempts to remediate visual neglect, modified from Luauté et al. (2006a). *VST* visual scanning training, *LA* limb activation, *rTMS* repetitive transcranial magnetic stimulation, *SAT* sustained attention training, *OPK* optokinetic, *NMV* neck muscle vibration, *TR* trunk rotation, *NA* noradrenergic agonists (Modified from Luauté et al. (2006a). © 2006, with permission from Elsevier)

the deficit and the ability to maintain attention voluntarily towards the left side (Weinberg et al. 1977; Gouvier et al. 1987; Antonucci et al. 1995), they do not always allow a generalization to daily life activities or to other tasks (Robertson et al. 1990). It has been proposed that the insufficient generalization of such techniques essentially based on endogenous attention depends on residual biases in exogenous attention in these patients (Seron et al. 1989).

9.2   Bottom-Up Techniques

At variance with top-down techniques, the following maneuvers do not require a high level of awareness of deficit or of voluntary control of attention to the left (Frassinetti et al. 2002). On the other hand, these maneuvers do not require or stimulate patients' active behavior. Perhaps as a consequence, lasting beneficial effects on neglect signs are confined to the approximate duration of sensory changes, so the improvement is usually limited in time and tends to disappear when the manipulation is interrupted (Chokron et al. 2007).

9.2.1   Vestibular Stimulation

Stimulation of vestibular nuclei can be achieved by using several techniques (Fig. 9.2). Caloric stimulation consists in introducing a small amount of cold water into an external auditory canal. Thermal energy conveyed through the temporal bone to the inner ear induces a convective flow of the endolymph, which in turn stimulates the vestibular sensors in the crista ampullaris of the semicircular canals (Lopez et al. 2012). This causes a deviation of the eyes and head in the direction of the irrigated ear.

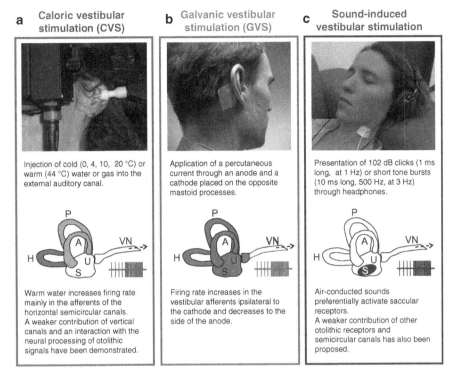

a Caloric vestibular stimulation (CVS)

Injection of cold (0, 4, 10, 20 °C) or warm (44 °C) water or gas into the external auditory canal.

Warm water increases firing rate mainly in the afferents of the horizontal semicircular canals. A weaker contribution of vertical canals and an interaction with the neural processing of otolithic signals have been demonstrated.

b Galvanic vestibular stimulation (GVS)

Application of a percutaneous current through an anode and a cathode placed on the opposite mastoid processes.

Firing rate increases in the vestibular afferents ipsilateral to the cathode and decreases to the side of the anode.

c Sound-induced vestibular stimulation

Presentation of 102 dB clicks (1 ms long, at 1 Hz) or short tone bursts (10 ms long, 500 Hz, at 3 Hz) through headphones.

Air-conducted sounds preferentially activate saccular receptors. A weaker contribution of other otolithic receptors and semicircular canals has also been proposed.

Fig. 9.2 Three techniques of vestibular stimulation. (**a**) Caloric vestibular stimulation consists of irrigating the external auditory canal with warm or cold water or airflow. (**b**) Galvanic vestibular stimulation consists of applying a weak percutaneous current through an anode and a cathode placed over the opposite mastoid processes. (**c**) Auditory stimuli such as clicks and short tone bursts can also stimulate the vestibular receptors (Reproduced from Lopez et al. (2012). © 2012, with permission from Elsevier)

With cold water irrigation of the left ear, the ocular deviation assumes the form of a slow-phase leftward nystagmus. A similar, if less intense, deviation can be induced by introducing warm water into the contralateral ear. Rubens (1985) tested the effect of the vestibular caloric stimulation in 18 neglect patients and showed a substantial, if transient, reduction of neglect signs on line cancellation and reading. Subsequent studies have demonstrated similarly transient effects on other manifestations often associated with neglect, such as anosognosia (Cappa et al. 1987), imaginal neglect (Rode and Perenin 1994), or somatoparaphrenic delusion (Bisiach et al. 1991). A possible mechanism contributing to these effects of vestibular caloric stimulation is that leftward eye movements induced by the stimulation can, as it were, "drag" attention to the left part of physical or imagined space (Gainotti 1993; Chokron et al. 2007).

Other means to stimulate the vestibular system, which have been shown to alleviate neglect signs, include optokinetic stimulation (Pizzamiglio et al. 1990) and galvanic stimulation (Rorsman et al. 1999). Neuroimaging data on normal participants (Fink et al. 2003) suggest that the effect of galvanic stimulation on line bisection judgments (landmark task, see Sect. 5.3.1) depends on modifications of the activity of the right posterior parietal and right ventral premotor cortex.

Fig. 9.3 Schematic depiction
of leftward optokinetic
stimulation

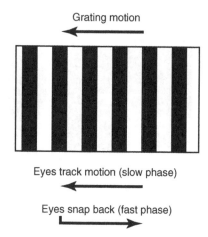

Optokinetic stimulation is based on a structured background (points or stripes) moving in a horizontal direction (Fig. 9.3). Optokinetic nystagmus occurs when looking at the moving stripes. Optokinetic nystagmus is also evoked by looking through the window of a moving train.

Pizzamiglio et al. (1990) demonstrated a decrease of line bisection error in neglect patients undergoing leftward optokinetic stimulation. However, in another experiment the same maneuver induced an increase of leftward error on the end-point task (see Sect. 5.3.2) (Bisiach et al. 1996). Bisiach et al. (1996) concluded that leftward optokinetic stimulation was able to mitigate neglect signs without acting directly on the underlying deficits.

9.2.2   Trunk Rotation

Karnath et al. (1993) obtained a reduction of signs of neglect by imposing a 15° leftward rotation of the trunk on left neglect patients. Based on this observation, Wiart et al. (1997) associated voluntary trunk rotation with visual exploration by means of a corset, to which a horizontal rod was attached. The rod allowed patients to point to colored figures placed on a panel in front of them (Fig. 9.4). Thus, patients were forced to produce an axial rotation of the torso in order to move the pointer sideways. During 20 1-h sessions, patients were trained to identify and reach the figures by using the rod. Wiart et al. (1997) observed positive effects of this procedure on neglect and daily living activities.

9.2.3   Mechanical and Electrical Transcutaneous Stimulations

Karnath et al. (1993) applied transcutaneous mechanical vibration to the muscles of the left side of the neck in left neglect patients during a lateralized visual detection

Fig. 9.4 The Bon Saint Côme device for coupling trunk rotation to visuospatial exploration (Reproduced from Wiart et al. (1997). © 1997, with permission from Elsevier)

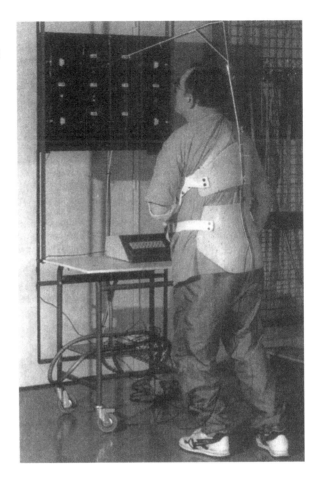

task and observed benefits similar to trunk rotation. Indeed, both maneuvers produce a lengthening of left posterior neck muscles (real with trunk rotation and apparent with mechanical stimulation). Vallar et al. (1995) used transcutaneous electrical neural stimulation, which also provides a somatosensory input to the vestibulo–proprioceptive system. When electrical stimulation was applied to the neck and the hand of neglect patients, there was a temporary improvement of neglect signs in most patients. Using this technique, Guariglia et al. (1998) were also able to improve imaginal neglect.

9.2.4 Stimulation of the Left Hand

This technique is based on the observation that signs of left neglect often decrease when the patient uses the left hand when performing standard paper-and-pencil tests (Halligan et al. 1991a). Robertson et al. (1992) have shown that this technique can reduce neglect in daily life for several weeks after the end of rehabilitation. Even a simple proprioceptive stimulation of the left hand can improve walking in patients (Robertson et al. 1994). Làdavas et al. (1997) found an improvement in a visual search task when passive movements of the left hand were performed in the left hemispace, while movements in the center or right or movements executed with the right hand did not ameliorate performance. These effects can occur for both near space and far space (Frassinetti et al. 2001).

9.2.5   Alertness Training

An important component deficit of neglect is impaired tonic alertness (see Sects. 1.2 and 6.2). As a consequence, stimulating phasic alerting with an acoustic tone can ameliorate visuospatial deficits in neglect (Robertson et al. 1998; Chica et al. 2012). On the other hand, in recovered patients a pharmacological challenge with a sedative GABAergic drug led to the reemergence of neglect signs (Lazar et al. 2002). Alertness training can also improve lateralized spatial deficits in brain-damaged patients by means of self-instructional (Robertson et al. 1995) or computerized methods (Sturm et al. 2006).

Thimm et al. (2006) explored the effects of a 3-week computerized alertness training on seven patients with chronic (>3 months) signs of neglect. There were improvements not only on alertness measures but also in the performance of a neglect test battery (see also Manly et al. (2005), and Fimm et al. (2006), for the effects of alertness in sleep-deprived healthy participants).

Functional MRI demonstrated that behavioral improvements were accompanied by an increase of BOLD responses in the frontal cortex, anterior cingulate cortex, precuneus, cuneus, and angular gyrus, in both hemispheres (Thimm et al. 2006). These areas have previously been associated with alertness and spatial attention (see Sects. 1.1 and 1.2). Unfortunately, behavioral improvements had receded 4 weeks after the end of the training, although the increases in neural activity bilaterally in frontal areas, in the right ACC, the right angular gyrus, and the left temporo-parietal cortex were still present.

DeGutis and Van Vleet (2010) trained patients with chronic neglect to frequently respond to nontarget stimuli and inhibit their response to infrequent, temporally unpredictable target stimuli for 36 min/day over 9 days. This task presumably engages both tonic and phasic alertness because patients have to employ endogenous alertness to perform the repetitive task of responding to the majority of the stimuli, whereas the infrequent, unpredictable target stimuli are likely to induce a strong phasic signal to inhibit a prepotent but inappropriate response. Trained patients improved on spatial and nonspatial measures of attention. In a follow-up experiment on three patients, the alertness training was compared to traditional search training and found to be more effective. Thus, training alertness might be a more effective treatment option in chronic neglect than direct training of spatial attention.

Fig. 9.5 Prismatic goggles
used for neglect rehabilitation

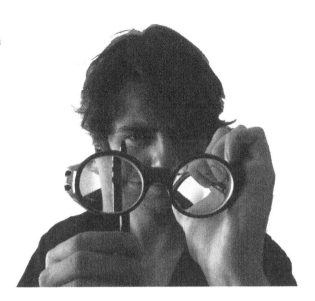

9.2.6   *Prism Adaptation*

Prism adaptation, first described by Rossetti et al. (1998), has been shown to improve neglect signs on both standard tests and functional scales. Patients are requested to make hand movements to reach a visual target while wearing optical prisms which deflect the entire visual field to the right (Fig. 9.5). After the prisms are removed, the same hand movements are performed.

While wearing the prisms, movements initially overshoot the target to the right because the visual system "sees" the target as displaced to the right of its actual position. After a few trials, patients learn to correct the initial movement overshooting (adaptation effect). After prisms are taken away, patients tend to overshoot left-ward of the actual target position (aftereffect). In the first study (Rossetti et al. 1998), after wearing prisms producing a 10° rightward visual deviation during 5 min, all patients displayed an adaptation effect, as well as an important aftereffect, consisting in a substantial, if transient, improvement of neglect signs.

Ensuing studies reported significant improvements in neglect signs after prism adaptation in a variety of situations: imaginal tasks (Rode et al. 1998, 2001), percep-tual tasks not involving arm movements (Farnè et al. 2002), moving in a wheelchair (Rossetti et al. 1999), and postural control tasks (Tilikete et al. 2001). Thus, the effect of prism adaptation is not only related to sensorimotor mechanisms, but it also influences cognitive processes (Mattingley 2002; Berberovic and Mattingley 2003; Rode et al. 2003). Regarding the duration of the effects induced by prism adaptation, Rossetti et al. (1998) observed an effect during two consecutive hours after adaptation; other studies have obtained positive effects for up to 1 week (Farnè et al. 2002). Frassinetti et al. (2002) had seven chronic neglect patients perform twice-daily sessions over a period of 2 weeks and observed long-lasting improvements, still present at a retest 5 weeks later.

A key advantage of prism adaptation over other techniques is that it requires only a short training period to produce lasting benefits (Frassinetti et al. 2002). Prism adaptation does not require voluntary orienting of attention towards the neglected side, at variance with other rehabilitation techniques for neglect (Angeli et al. 2004). The exact mechanisms underlying the effects of prism adaptation are unknown, although visuomotor transformations through cortico-cerebellar circuits are likely to play a role (Luaute et al. 2006b).

9.3 Noninvasive Brain Stimulation

Noninvasive brain stimulation techniques, including transcranial magnetic stimulation (TMS) and transcranial direct current stimulation (tDCS), are promising techniques for modulating human cognition, although the possible costs of such modulations are yet to be established (Brem et al. 2013). The mechanisms of action of these techniques are not yet fully understood, but it is widely accepted that they can modulate the level of cortical excitability in specific neural networks, including the attention networks.

TMS has been used to modulate the interhemispheric interactions in left neglect. Interference on the parietal cortex in the left, unaffected hemisphere (Fig. 9.6) has repeatedly been shown to ameliorate signs of left neglect.

For example, Oliveri et al. (2001) applied repetitive 1 Hz TMS on the unaffected hemisphere in two left-brain-damaged and five right-brain-damaged patients and obtained a transient decrease of neglect on the landmark task. Brighina et al. (2003) treated three right-brain-damaged patients with left neglect by administering 900 pulses (1 Hz frequency) over the left PPC every other day for 2 weeks. Patients showed improved performance on the landmark task, which remained unchanged 2 weeks after the end of the stimulation cycle and which was also generalized to other neglect tests. Relatively durable effects (up to 32 h) on perception of left-sided stimuli were obtained by Nyffeler et al. (2009), by using a single-day application of theta-burst TMS with 11 right-brain-damaged patients with left neglect.

Koch et al. (2012) performed a rigorous double-blind trial of the effect of theta-burst TMS stimulation on the left parietal region of patients with right hemisphere damage and signs of left visual neglect. Neglect improved in stimulated patients more than in those receiving sham TMS. Real, but not sham, TMS also decreased motor cortex excitability in the left hemisphere, thus providing an important supporting result, consistent with the hypothesis that signs of left neglect may in part result from hyperactivity of the left hemisphere (but see Sect. 6.1.6).

Müri et al. (2013) reviewed ten studies that used TMS for neglect rehabilitation and two studies that used another noninvasive stimulation technique, tDCS. They concluded that while evidence on efficacy of these stimulations is still uncertain, results are promising especially for theta-burst stimulation and suggest that TMS can be a powerful adjuvant therapy in the rehabilitation of neglect patients.

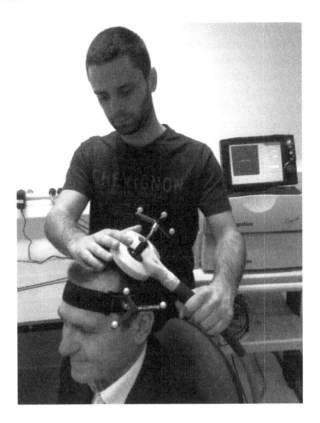

Fig. 9.6 Transcranial magnetic stimulation of the left parietal lobe

9.4 Pharmacological Treatments

Several drugs have been attempted to ameliorate neglect, mainly acting on dopaminergic, noradrenergic, or cholinergic systems. Since different drugs act on receptors differently distributed in the central nervous system, lesion anatomy can be a predictor of response to specific drugs in individual patients (Coulthard et al. 2006). For the moment, however, pharmacological treatment of neglect remains largely in the research domain and has not yet translated into clinical practice.

9.4.1 Dopaminergic Agents

Over the past few decades, various drugs modulating dopaminergic activity have been used in single case reports or small groups of neglect patients with variable results, including occasional worsening of neglect signs. Improvements were described with apomorphine (Geminiani et al. 1998), levodopa (Mukand et al. 2001), or bromocriptine (Fleet et al. 1987), but not with amantadine (Buxbaum et al. 2007). In other reports, however, bromocriptine negatively affected neglect (Grujic et al. 1998; Barrett et al. 1999).

More recently, Gorgoraptis et al. (2012) conducted a double-blind, randomized, placebo-controlled trial with rotigotine, an agonist with prevalent D1 activity. In the monkey, the activity of D1 receptors in the PFC is important for spatial working memory (Williams and Goldman-Rakic 1995), which can be impaired in neglect (see Sect. 6.4.1). D1 activity has also been shown to modulate attention and alertness (Bromberg-Martin et al. 2010), whose impairment can also contribute to neglect. Gorgoraptis et al. (2012) used a clever statistical procedure, which permitted the treatment of each patient as his/her own control. As a consequence, the results are statistically solid even for relatively small sample sizes ($n = 16$ in this case). Results showed a moderate but significant improvement related to rotigotine on a visual search task. Unfortunately, contrary to the predictions the improvement did not seem to affect spatial working memory performance or to correlate with the degree of damage to the right PFC.

9.4.2 Noradrenergic Agents

Noradrenergic projections from the locus coeruleus to the cortex are important to maintain vigilance during task performance (see Sect. 1.2 above).

The [alpha]2A-noradrenergic agonist guanfacine has been used in a small double-blind study (Malhotra et al. 2006) with three neglect patients, two of whom showed some improvement on a visual search task. The patient who did not respond to guanfacine had extensive damage to the right dorsolateral PFC, a possible target structure for the drug.

9.4.3 Cholinergic Agents

Cholinergic activity modulates alertness and other attention processes through diffuse projections from the basal forebrain to frontoparietal and sensory areas (Sarter and Bruno 1999).

The cholinergic agonist nicotine has been shown to facilitate several subcomponents of attention reorienting via modulation of inferior parietal, temporal, and frontal brain activity in the right hemisphere (Thiel and Fink 2008). Lucas et al. (2013) explored the effect of a single dose (10 mg) of transdermal nicotine patch on spatial neglect in ten stroke patients in a double-blind placebo-controlled protocol. Nicotine improved patients' performance on cancellation tasks and facilitated orienting to single visual targets, but had no significant effect on other tests. Lucas et al. (2013) concluded that nicotine had a global effect on attention and alertness, but no effect on space-based deficits in neglect.

Acetylcholinesterase inhibitors, such as donepezil (Berthier et al. 2006) or rivastigmine (Paolucci et al. 2010), have been proposed to accelerate recovery from neuropsychological deficits after stroke. In one study, rivastigmine led to better neglect scores at discharge, but at 1-month follow-up nontreated patients had reached a similar level of recovery as the treated group (Paolucci et al. 2010).

References

Angeli V, Meneghello F, Mattioli F, Ladavas E. Mechanisms underlying visuo-spatial amelioration of neglect after prism adaptation. Cortex. 2004;40:155–6.

Antonucci G, Guariglia C, Judica A, Magnotti L, Paolucci S, Pizzamiglio L, Zoccolotti P. Effectiveness of neglect rehabilitation in a randomized group study. J Clin Exp Neuropsychol. 1995;17:383–9.

Barrett AM, Crucian GP, Schwartz RL, Heilman KM. Adverse effect of dopamine agonist therapy in a patient with motor-intentional neglect. Arch Phys Med Rehabil. 1999;80:600–3.

Berberovic N, Mattingley JB. Effects of prismatic adaptation on judgments of spatial extent in peripersonal and extrapersonal space. Neuropsychologia. 2003;41:493–503.

Berthier ML, Green C, Higueras C, Fernandez I, Hinojosa J, Martin MC. A randomized, placebo-controlled study of donepezil in poststroke aphasia. Neurology. 2006;67:1687–9.

Bisiach E, Rusconi ML, Vallar G. Remission of somatoparaphrenic delusion through vestibular stimulation. Neuropsychologia. 1991;29:1029–31.

Bisiach E, Pizzamiglio L, Nico D, Antonucci G. Beyond unilateral neglect. Brain. 1996;119:851–7.

Brem A-K, Fried PJ, Horvath JC, Robertson EM, Pascual-Leone A. Is neuroenhancement by noninvasive brain stimulation a net zero-sum proposition? Neuroimage. 2013.

Brighina F, Bisiach E, Oliveri M, Piazza A, La Bua V, Daniele O, Fierro B. 1 Hz repetitive transcranial magnetic stimulation of the unaffected hemisphere ameliorates contralesional visuospatial neglect in humans. Neurosci Lett. 2003;336:131–3.

Bromberg-Martin ES, Matsumoto M, Hikosaka O. Dopamine in motivational control: rewarding, aversive, and alerting. Neuron. 2010;68:815–34.

Buxbaum LJ, Ferraro M, Whyte J, Gershkoff A, Coslett HB. Amantadine treatment of hemispatial neglect: a double-blind, placebo-controlled study. Am J Phys Med Rehabil. 2007;86:527–37.

Cappa SF, Sterzi R, Vallar G, Bisiach E. Remission of hemineglect and anosognosia during vestibular stimulation. Neuropsychologia. 1987;25:775–82.

Chica AB, Thiebaut de Schotten M, Toba MN, Malhotra P, Lupiáñez J, Bartolomeo P. Attention networks and their interactions after right-hemisphere damage. Cortex. 2012;48:654–63.

Chokron S, Dupierrix E, Tabert M, Bartolomeo P. Experimental remission of unilateral spatial neglect. Neuropsychologia. 2007;45:3127–48.

Coulthard E, Singh-Curry V, Husain M. Treatment of attention deficits in neurological disorders. Curr Opin Neurol. 2006;19:613–8.

DeGutis JM, Van Vleet TM. Tonic and phasic alertness training: a novel behavioral therapy to improve spatial and non-spatial attention in patients with hemispatial neglect. Front Hum Neurosci. 2010;4:60.

Farnè A, Rossetti Y, Toniolo S, Ladavas E. Ameliorating neglect with prism adaptation: visuo-manual and visuo-verbal measures. Neuropsychologia. 2002;40:718–29.

Fimm B, Willmes K, Spijkers W. The effect of low arousal on visuo-spatial attention. Neuropsychologia. 2006;44:1261–8.

Fink GR, Marshall JC, Weiss PH, Stephan T, Grefkes C, Shah NJ, Zilles K, Dieterich M. Performing allocentric visuospatial judgments with induced distortion of the egocentric reference frame: an fMRI study with clinical implications. Neuroimage. 2003;20:1505–17.

Fleet WS, Valenstein E, Watson RT, Heilman KM. Dopamine agonist therapy for neglect in humans. Neurology. 1987;37:1765–70.

Frassinetti F, Rossi M, Làdavas E. Passive limb movements improve visual neglect. Neuropsychologia. 2001;39:725–33.

Frassinetti F, Angeli V, Meneghello F, Avanzi S, Ladavas E. Long-lasting amelioration of visuo-spatial neglect by prism adaptation. Brain. 2002;125:608–23.

Gainotti G. The role of spontaneous eye movements in orienting attention and in unilateral neglect. In: Robertson IH, Marshall JC, editors. Unilateral neglect: clinical and experimental studies. Hove: Lawrence Erlbaum Associates; 1993. p. 107–22.

Geminiani G, Bottini G, Sterzi R. Dopaminergic stimulation in unilateral neglect. J Neurol Neurosurg Psychiatry. 1998;65:344–7.

Gorgoraptis N, Mah YH, Machner B, Singh-Curry V, Malhotra P, Hadji-Michael M, Cohen D, Simister R, Nair A, Kulinskaya E, Ward N, Greenwood R, Husain M. The effects of the dopamine agonist rotigotine on hemispatial neglect following stroke. Brain. 2012;135:2478–91.

Gouvier W, Bua B, Blanton P, Urey J. Behavioural changes following visual scanning training: observations of five cases. Int J Clin Neuropsychol. 1987;9:74–80.

Grujic Z, Mapstone M, Gitelman DR, Johnson N, Weintraub S, Hays A, Kwasnica C, Harvey R, Mesulam MM. Dopamine agonists reorient visual exploration away from the neglected hemispace. Neurology. 1998;51:1395–8.

Guariglia C, Lippolis G, Pizzamiglio L. Somatosensory stimulation improves imagery disorders in neglect. Cortex. 1998;34:233–41.

Halligan PW, Bartolomeo P. Visual neglect. In: Ramachandran VS, editor. Encyclopedia of human behavior. 2nd ed. vol. 3. San Diego: Academic Press; 2012. p. 652–64.

Halligan PW, Manning L, Marshall JC. Hemispheric activation vs spatio-motor cuing in visual neglect: a case study. Neuropsychologia. 1991;29:165–76.

Karnath H-O, Christ K, Hartje W. Decrease of contralateral neglect by neck muscle vibration and spatial orientation of trunk midline. Brain. 1993;116:383–96.

Koch G, Bonni S, Giacobbe V, Bucchi G, Basile B, Lupo F, Versace V, Bozzali M, Caltagirone C. Theta-burst stimulation of the left hemisphere accelerates recovery of hemispatial neglect. Neurology. 2012;78:24–30.

Làdavas E, Berti A, Ruozzi E, Barboni F. Neglect as a deficit determined by an imbalance between multiple spatial representations. Exp Brain Res. 1997;116:493–500.

Lazar RM, Fitzsimmons B-F, Marshall RS, Berman MF, Bustillo MA, Young WL, Mohr JP, Shah J, Robinson JV. Reemergence of stroke deficits with midazolam challenge. Stroke. 2002;33:283–5.

Lopez C, Blanke O, Mast FW. The human vestibular cortex revealed by coordinate-based activation likelihood estimation meta-analysis. Neuroscience. 2012;212:159–79.

Luaute J, Halligan P, Rode G, Rossetti Y, Boisson D. Visuo-spatial neglect: a systematic review of current interventions and their effectiveness. Neurosci Biobehav Rev. 2006a;30:961–82.

Luaute J, Michel C, Rode G, Pisella L, Jacquin-Courtois S, Costes N, Cotton F, le Bars D, Boisson D, Halligan P, Rossetti Y. Functional anatomy of the therapeutic effects of prism adaptation on left neglect. Neurology. 2006b;66:1859–67.

Lucas N, Saj A, Schwartz S, Ptak R, Thomas C, Conne P, Leroy R, Pavin S, Diserens K, Vuilleumier P. Effects of pro-cholinergic treatment in patients suffering from spatial neglect. Front Hum Neurosci. 2013;7:574.

Malhotra PA, Parton AD, Greenwood R, Husain M. Noradrenergic modulation of space exploration in visual neglect. Ann Neurol. 2006;59:186–90.

Manly T, Dobler VB, Dodds CM, George MA. Rightward shift in spatial awareness with declining alertness. Neuropsychologia. 2005;43:1721–8.

Mattingley JB. Visuomotor adaptation to optical prisms: a new cure for spatial neglect? Cortex. 2002;38:277–83.

Mukand JA, Guilmette TJ, Allen DG, Brown LK, Brown SL, Tober KL, Vandyck WR. Dopaminergic therapy with carbidopa L-dopa for left neglect after stroke: a case series. Arch Phys Med Rehabil. 2001;82:1279–82.

Müri RM, Cazzoli D, Nef T, Mosimann UP, Hopfner S, Nyffeler T. Non-invasive brain stimulation in neglect rehabilitation: an update. Front Hum Neurosci. 2013;7:248.

Nyffeler T, Cazzoli D, Hess CW, Müri RM. One session of repeated parietal theta burst stimulation trains induces long-lasting improvement of visual neglect. Stroke. 2009;40:2791–6.

Oliveri M, Bisiach E, Brighina F, Piazza A, La Bua V, Buffa D, Fierro B. RTMS of the unaffected hemisphere transiently reduces contralesional visuospatial hemineglect. Neurology. 2001;57:1338–40.

Paolucci S, Bureca I, Multari M, Nocentini U, Matano A. An open-label pilot study of the use of rivastigmine to promote functional recovery in patients with unilateral spatial neglect due to first ischemic stroke. Funct Neurol. 2010;25:195–200.

Pizzamiglio L, Frasca R, Guariglia C, Incoccia C, Antonucci G. Effect of optokinetic stimulation in patients with visual neglect. Cortex. 1990;26:535–40.

Robertson IH, Gray JM, Pentland B, Waite LJ. Microcomputer-based rehabilitation for unilateral left visual neglect: a randomized controlled trial. Arch Phys Med Rehabil. 1990;71:663–8.

Robertson IH, North NT, Geggie C. Spatio-motor cueing in unilateral left neglect: three case studies of its therapeutic effects. J Neurol Neurosurg Psychiatry. 1992;55:799–805.

Robertson IH, Tegner R, Goodrich SJ, Wilson C. Walking trajectory and hand movements in unilateral left neglect: a vestibular hypothesis. Neuropsychologia. 1994;32:1495–502.

Robertson IH, Tegner R, Tham K, Lo A, Nimmo-Smith I. Sustained attention training for unilateral neglect: theoretical and rehabilitation implications. J Clin Exp Neuropsychol. 1995;17:416–30.

Robertson IH, Mattingley JB, Rorden C, Driver J. Phasic alerting of neglect patients overcomes their spatial deficit in visual awareness. Nature. 1998;395:169–72.

Rode G, Perenin MT. Temporary remission of representational hemineglect through vestibular stimulation. NeuroReport. 1994;5:869–72.

Rode G, Rossetti Y, Li L, Boisson D. The effect of prism adaptation on neglect for visual imagery. Behav Neurol. 1998;11:251–8.

Rode G, Rossetti Y, Boisson D. Prism adaptation improves representational neglect. Neuropsychologia. 2001;39:1250–4.

Rode G, Pisella L, Rossetti Y, Farnè A, Boisson D. Bottom-up transfer of sensory-motor plasticity to recovery of spatial cognition: visuomotor adaptation and spatial neglect. Prog Brain Res. 2003;142:273–87.

Rorsman I, Magnusson M, Johansson BB. Reduction of visuo-spatial neglect with vestibular galvanic stimulation. Scand J Rehabil Med. 1999;31:117–24.

Rossetti Y, Rode G, Pisella L, Farnè A, Li L, Boisson D, Perenin MT. Prism adaptation to a rightward optical deviation rehabilitates left hemispatial neglect. Nature. 1998;395:166–9.

Rossetti Y, Rode G, Boisson D. Sensori-motor plasticity and the rehabilitation of hemispatial neglect (plasticité sensori-motrice et récupération fonctionnelle: les effets thérapeutiques de l'adaptation prismatique sur la négligence spatiale unilatérale). Medecine/Sciences. 1999;15:239–45.

Rubens AB. Caloric stimulation and unilateral visual neglect. Neurology. 1985;35:1019–24.

Sarter M, Bruno JP. Cortical cholinergic inputs mediating arousal, attentional processing and dreaming: differential afferent regulation of the basal forebrain by telencephalic and brainstem afferents. Neuroscience. 1999;95:933–52.

Seron X, Deloche G, Coyette F. A retrospective analysis of a single case neglect therapy: a point of theory. In: Seron X, Deloche G, editors. Cognitive approaches in neuropsychological rehabilitation. Hillsdale: Lawrence Erlbaum Associates; 1989. p. 289–316.

Sturm W, Thimm M, Kust J, Karbe H, Fink GR. Alertness-training in neglect: behavioral and imaging results. Restor Neurol Neurosci. 2006;24:371–84.

Thiel CM, Fink GR. Effects of the cholinergic agonist nicotine on reorienting of visual spatial attention and top-down attentional control. Neuroscience. 2008;152:381–90.

Thimm M, Fink GR, Kust J, Karbe H, Sturm W. Impact of alertness training on spatial neglect: a behavioural and fMRI study. Neuropsychologia. 2006;44:1230–46.

Tilikete C, Rode G, Rossetti Y, Li L, Pichon J, Boisson D. Prism adaptation to rightward optical deviation improves postural imbalance in left hemiparetic patients. Curr Biol. 2001;11:524–8.

Vallar G, Rusconi ML, Barozzi S, Bernardini B, Ovadia D, Papagno C, Cesarini A. Improvement of left visuo-spatial hemineglect by left-sided transcutaneous electrical stimulation. Neuropsychologia. 1995;33:73–82.

Weinberg J, Diller J, Gordon WA, Gerstman LJ, Lieberman A, Lakin P, Hodges G, Ezrachi O. Visual scanning training effect on reading-related tasks in acquired right-brain damage. Arch Phys Med Rehabil. 1977;58:479–86.

Wiart L, Bon Saint Come A, Debelleix X, Petit H, Joseph PA, Mazaux JM, Barat M. Unilateral neglect syndrome rehabilitation by trunk rotation and scanning training. Arch Phys Med Rehabil. 1997;78:424–9.

Williams GV, Goldman-Rakic PS. Modulation of memory fields by dopamine D1 receptors in prefrontal cortex. Nature. 1995;376:572–5.

Further Reading

Coulthard E, Singh-Curry V, Husain M. Treatment of attention deficits in neurological disorders. Curr Opin Neurol. 2006;19:613–8.

Halligan PW, Bartolomeo P. Visual neglect. In: Ramachandran VS, editor. Encyclopedia of human behavior. 2nd ed. vol. 3. San Diego: Academic; 2012. p. 652–64.

Luaute J, Halligan P, Rode G, Rossetti Y, Boisson D. Visuo-spatial neglect: a systematic review of current interventions and their effectiveness. Neurosci Biobehav Rev. 2006;30:961–82.

Müri RM, Cazzoli D, Nef T, Mosimann UP, Hopfner S, Nyffeler T. Non-invasive brain stimulation in neglect rehabilitation: an update. Front Hum Neurosci. 2013;7:248.

Conclusion and Perspectives

The main aim of this volume was to provide a mostly clinical guide to a range of neuropsychological deficits which typically result from right hemisphere damage. Most of these deficits have a connection, more or less direct, with impaired attention processes. Some of these processes appear to have a tight, if not completely understood, relationship with the right hemisphere in most normal dextrals.

A fascinating hypothesis holds that hemispheric specialization was already in place when vertebrates arose 500 million years ago (MacNeilage et al. 2009). The left hemisphere might originally have focused on controlling well-established patterns of behavior, hence its specialization in speech and manipulation (right-handedness). The right hemisphere, on the other hand, would have specialized early in detecting and responding to unexpected stimuli, in order to quickly detect predators. This division of labor would thus have assigned processes dedicated to fast detection, such as face recognition, attention processes, and spatial cognition, mainly to the right hemisphere. The functional and anatomical asymmetries of the human brain, as well as the consequences of unilateral hemispheric lesions, seem broadly consistent with this view, although experiments on monkeys have hitherto failed to provide evidence of hemispheric lateralization of attention functions similar to those occurring in the human brain. These considerations underline the importance of the right hemisphere to "put us in our place in the world," as the late professor Jean-Denis Degos used to say.

What evidence from brain-damaged patients clearly indicates is that attention processes, mainly subserved by frontoparietal brain networks, with a special although not yet completely elucidated role for the right hemisphere, enable us to be aware of our own body and to actively explore the external world. Attention impairments such as those resulting from right brain damage can hamper the patients' conscious perception of objects in space and of their own limbs and are a substantial source of handicap and disability.

The clinical reality of these patients provides an important teaching for the cognitive neuroscience of perception: neurological patients who do not explore a portion of their visual environment, as a consequence of attention disorders, can be far more handicapped in their daily life than patients with sensory deficits affecting

P. Bartolomeo, *Attention Disorders After Right Brain Damage*,
DOI 10.1007/978-1-4471-5649-9, © Springer-Verlag London 2014

perception directly but leaving attention unimpaired, such as decreased visual acuity or homonymous hemianopia.

It is easy to anticipate that the models of attention processes, used here to tentatively frame the multiform empirical evidence resulting from patients' patterns of behavior, are likely to be recast, with time, into new and perhaps completely different theoretical frameworks, such as models addressing how the brain minimizes prediction errors in an uncertain environment (Clark 2013).

Unfortunately, our present knowledge of the brain attention systems is not yet adequate to enable us to always offer specific interventions for the attention disorders described herein. However, a major successful outcome of research in the last decade has been the discovery that attention disorders are not so much related to damage of cortical modules, as to complex patterns of dysfunction in large-scale brain networks. There are far-reaching scientific and clinical implications of this important finding, which are only beginning to surface. Cognitive neuroscience needs to rebuild its localist models on the much more complex scale of network interactions. Patient management is now starting to benefit from the possibility to act on the undamaged nodes of the attention networks.

With the neuroscientific pursuit of such objectives and as clinical research continues in search of long-term improvements of patients' conditions, our earnest hope is that a growing understanding of these conditions, with the consequent development of effective methods to diagnose and manage neurological patients with attention disorders, will, in time, render many of the more tentative conclusions of this book outdated.

References

Clark A. Whatever next? Predictive brains, situated agents, and the future of cognitive science. Behav Brain Sci. 2013;36:181–204.

MacNeilage PF, Rogers LJ, Vallortigara G. Origins of the left & right brain. Sci Am. 2009; 301:60–7.

Subject Index

P. Bartolomeo, *Attention Disorders After Right Brain Damage*,
DOI 10.1007/978-1-4471-5649-9, © Springer-Verlag London 2014

Author Index

Lightning Source UK Ltd.
Milton Keynes UK
UKOW06n1319250416

272925UK00002B/4/P